NREMT STUDY STUDY GUIDE

2024-2025

Achieving EMT Certification Success | A Comprehensive
Preparation Resource with 800 Test Questions,
In-Depth Strategies, and Essential Tips

VERE SIMONDS

TABLE OF CONTENTS

INTRODUCTION

The Importance of EMT Certification

Becoming an Emergency Medical Technician, commonly known as an EMT, is one of the boldest steps you can take towards serving your community. As the first responder in most emergency medical situations, an EMT plays a crucial role in providing immediate care to those in urgent need. If you're considering this career path or are simply curious about it, understanding the significance of EMT certification is essential.

EMT certification serves as an endorsement of your expertise, confirming that you have met national standards for the knowledge and skills necessary to provide prehospital emergency medical care. It's like having a badge that tells patients, co-workers, and employers, *"I've got this."* You don't just wake up one day and decide to be an EMT; you work hard for it.

The journey to becoming a certified EMT begins with education. You enroll in an EMT course that must be accredited. This ensures that what you're learning is not only up-to-date but also relevant and standardized across the board. These courses cover everything from basic first aid skills to more complex procedures like assessing patients and dealing with traumatic injuries. There's plenty of hands-on practice too so that when you're out there in the field, it's not all new to you.

But why is this certification so important? First off, it's evidence that you're capable of doing the job correctly. Think about it — in emergencies, every second count. The care provided by EMTs can mean the difference between life and death. By completing your certification, you show that you can make these critical decisions quickly and execute procedures effectively under stress.

EMT certification also includes passing cognitive and psychomotor exams. The cognitive exam tests your understanding of emergency care fundamentals through questions on medical emergencies, cardiology, trauma, and more. The psychomotor exam puts your hands-on abilities to the test—everything from patient assessment to managing cardiac arrest scenarios.

Another aspect is credibility. As a certified EMT, trust gets placed upon you both legally and ethically to handle medical situations appropriately. It signals to others that you abide by a strict code of conduct and adhere to protocols set by medical authorities.

Let's not forget about employment opportunities. Certification is frequently required by employers before they even consider letting you through their doors for an interview. In many places, it's actually illegal to practice as an EMT without proper certification due to the potential risks involved.

Continuous education is another component tied closely with certification. As medical practices evolve and new technologies emerge, ongoing training ensures that EMTs stay knowledgeable about the latest advances in emergency medicine. This further attests to why maintaining certification through continued education is vital—it keeps your skills sharp and your knowledge fresh.

How to Use This Study Guide

This study guide is meticulously crafted to help you navigate the challenging yet rewarding path toward EMT certification, a crucial milestone for anyone passionate about delivering urgent medical care in diverse settings. As you embark on this educational adventure, it's paramount to grasp the significance of achieving EMT certification. It stands as a testament to your dedication, competencies, and readiness to serve those in need. Furthermore, it is a pivotal step in securing a vital role within the emergency medical services (EMS) system, where your actions can mean the difference between life and death.

This guide provides an expansive array of resources designed to prepare you for the National Registry Emergency Medical Technician (NREMT) exam. Understanding your role and responsibilities sets the foundation for your training. You will learn about the legal and ethical frameworks that govern EMS practice and explore how to maintain workplace safety and personal wellness amidst the challenges of emergency care.

Preparatory knowledge forms the backbone of effective EMT practice. Through this guide, you will delve into the intricacies of human anatomy and physiology, equip yourself with basic pathophysiological principles, and gain insight into pharmacology tailored for EMT usage.

Mastering patient assessment is critical; you must be adept at conducting thorough scene size-ups, primary and secondary assessments, and utilizing vital signs and monitoring devices efficiently.

Airway management could not be more central to emergency care; recognizing airway anatomy and physiology allows you to manage airway obstructions effectively and understand ventilation devices alongside oxygen delivery systems.

Cardiology encompasses skills such as managing cardiovascular emergencies, using automated external defibrillators, and performing cardiopulmonary resuscitation across all age groups. Medical emergencies extend beyond cardiology; thus, we cover strategies for medical assessment and managing common medical scenarios, including obstetrical emergencies and childbirth.

Trauma care brings its unique set of challenges. You'll learn about trauma assessment management, controlling bleeding, shock management, addressing soft tissue injuries, as well as musculoskeletal damage.

Caring for infants and children demands special knowledge; our guide ensures you're well-versed in pediatric care by covering assessment techniques specific to young patients alongside frequently encountered pediatric emergencies. Operations are integral too; principles of EMS operations introduce concepts such as incident management across multiple-casualty events along with ground and air ambulance operations.

Moreover, advanced preparation techniques equip you with study strategies, memory aids, mnemonics, plus time management tools to efficiently prepare for the NREMT exam. To test your readiness, full-length practice exams are provided with explanations for each answer.

Lastly, you'll find invaluable advice on test-taking strategies aimed at mitigating anxiety and stress while maximizing exam performance. Post-exam guidance assists in interpreting results if needed while providing strategies should you need a retake. Transitioning from student to EMT professional is demystified as we also look ahead to continuing education opportunities for professional growth within EMS.

The journey ahead is demanding but immensely fulfilling. With this guide in hand, your readiness for achieving EMT certification success is assured. Let us begin this transformative process together!

CHAPTER 1
EMT ROLE AND RESPONSIBILITIES

The EMT scope of practice includes a range of skills that are essential for providing immediate, lifesaving interventions while awaiting additional EMS resources to arrive. It also involves non-life-threatening care and transport, with the primary focus being on patient safety and comfort.

EMTs are trained to assess a patient's condition and manage respiratory, cardiac, and trauma emergencies. However, their role does not end with prehospital care; they serve as crucial communicators during the transfer of patients to emergency departments or other healthcare facilities.

Imagine an EMT as a first responder during various emergencies – whether it is a road accident, natural disaster, or health crisis like a heart attack or stroke. They quickly evaluate the situation using their training on assessing patient needs. This initial assessment includes checking airway, breathing and circulation (often noted as ABCs) and making sure the environment is safe for themselves and others.

After assessment, EMTs may provide life-saving treatment such as CPR (cardiopulmonary resuscitation), use automated external defibrillators (AEDs), administer oxygen or perform basic interventions like controlling bleeding by applying bandages or using tourniquets.

They are also trained to assist in childbirth situations and provide support for patients experiencing mental health crises.

An essential part of their role is documentation; during and after emergency care has been given, EMTs must record their assessments and treatments accurately. This information is crucial for ongoing care at medical facilities.

While EMTs are trained in many procedures, there are limitations on what they can do legally within their scope of practice – defined by state regulations which vary from one area to another. For instance, they can't perform tasks that require advanced training like administering most medications or invasive procedures - those are the domain of more advanced practitioners like Paramedics.

Legal and Ethical Considerations

Every medical professional must operate within ethical and legal standards; EMTs are no exception. They must always prioritize patient care while maintaining professional behavior.

On the legal side of things, an important concept that every EMT must watch out for is consent. Patients have the right to either accept or refuse treatment; it's up to the EMT to get this consent unless a person can't provide it due to their condition (usually we refer to this as implied consent). If an awake patient says 'no' to treatment or transport despite needing it urgently, an EMT must respect this decision but also try explaining why receiving treatment is crucial for their health.

Confidentiality is another significant legal concern. Personal information about a patient's health status must be guarded closely according to laws like HIPAA (Health Insurance Portability & Accountability Act) in the United States which protects patient privacy.

Alongside legal considerations are ethical ones – for instance maintaining trust by being honest with patients about their conditions without causing unnecessary distress. This includes being sensitive towards different cultural beliefs patients may have about treatments or procedures.

Moreover, it's ethically important not to judge patients based on who they are or what situation they might be in - providing fair care regardless of age, gender, race also goes for socioeconomic status and more.

In all cases where tough decisions have to be made swiftly in chaotic emergency settings – knowing legal boundaries while sticking firm on ethical high ground guides an EMT's actions towards doing what's best for a patient.

Workplace Safety and Wellness

Without a doubt, your safety and wellness are central to being effective in your role as an EMT. It's imperative that you follow established safety procedures to protect yourself from potential hazards like bloodborne pathogens or dangerous scenes such as fire ground operations or road traffic accidents. Infection control is a critical component of workplace safety. You'll be trained in the use of personal protective equipment (PPE), such as gloves or eye protection when dealing with blood or bodily fluids—to reduce the risk of contracting or spreading diseases.

Another aspect is mental wellness. Facing high-stress conditions on a daily basis can take a toll on your mental health. Being proactive about stress management through debriefings after intense calls or taking advantage of counseling services is essential in maintaining your wellbeing.

Good physical fitness also plays a role in your ability to perform the job well; thus regular exercise and proper nutrition should be part of your routine to ensure you're always ready to respond to emergencies. Lastly, one often overlooked aspect of wellness is sleep. While shift work can disrupt normal sleep patterns, strive for adequate rest to keep your mind clear and body prepared for the physical demands of the job.

CHAPTER 2
PREPARATORY KNOWLEDGE

The Human Body and Systems

The human body is an amazing structure, made up of many different systems that work together to keep us alive and well. Understanding these systems is vital for anyone interested in emergency medical response. Let's look at the key systems one by one.

The **circulatory system** is like a transportation network, with the heart as its engine. The heart pumps blood through a series of pipes, or blood vessels, which carry nutrients and oxygen to every part of the body. This system also carries away waste products. Blood is composed of different parts, including red blood cells that carry oxygen, white blood cells that fight infections, and platelets that help with clotting when we get hurt.

Next is the **respiratory system**. Think of this as our air supply. It allows us to breathe by taking in oxygen from the air and getting rid of carbon dioxide we don't need. The key players are the nose, throat, voice box, windpipe, and lungs. When we breathe in air through our nose or mouth, it travels down the windpipe and into our two lungs. Here, oxygen is passed into the blood and carbon dioxide is taken from the blood and breathed out.

Our **digestive system** has an important job: breaking down food so our body can use it for energy. It starts in the mouth with chewing and mixes food with spit to make it soft. The food then goes down a tube called the esophagus into our stomach, where it gets mixed more. Food moves next into our intestines where nutrients are absorbed into the bloodstream and waste moves onwards to be removed from our body.

The **skeletal system** gives our body structure – it's like our internal framework made of bones. Bones come in all sizes and serve many roles such as protecting organs (like the brain inside our skull), supporting weight (like legs holding us up), and allowing movement (like arms swinging). Together with muscles - part of muscular system - they help us move around.

Muscles are powerful tissues that contract (shorten) and relax to create movement. There are over 600 muscles working with bones to walk, lift things, pump blood through our heart – pretty much any movement you can think of. They also produce heat to keep our bodies at a stable temperature.

The **nervous system** is like the command center or computer network that controls everything we do – both voluntary actions like walking or involuntary ones like breathing. It uses electrical signals to send messages around your body through a network of nerves connected to your brain and spinal cord.

Another important system is the **endocrine system** which sends out chemicals called hormones into our bloodstream to control various functions such as growth or responding to stress. Our **urinary system** cleans up by filtering out waste from our blood into urine which we then get rid of when we go to the restroom. The kidneys are star players here; they filter waste and extra fluid not needed by your body.

Lastly, let's not forget about skin which is part of your **integumentary system**; it protects everything inside you from infections and injuries while also helping control body temperature.

From providing nutrients to fighting off diseases, these systems keep things running smoothly under most conditions so understanding them helps anyone prepare better for emergencies where things might not be going as they should within someone's body.

Basics of Pathophysiology

Pathophysiology is the study of how disease processes affect the function of the body. It's an essential area of knowledge for anyone in the medical field, especially for those studying to become emergency medical technicians (EMTs). Understanding pathophysiology allows you to recognize how diseases and injuries interact with the body's systems and processes.

In our bodies, the normal physiological state is called homeostasis. This is when everything is functioning optimally, and the internal environment is balanced. However, when we encounter pathogens, suffer from genetic anomalies, or endure injuries, our bodies may enter a state of dysfunction—this is where pathophysiology begins.

Let's start by looking at how the body responds to injury or infection. The inflammatory response is critical here. When tissues are damaged, the body releases chemicals that cause blood vessels to leak fluid into the tissues, resulting in swelling. This inflammation allows for more immune cells to travel to the site of injury or infection and often causes redness and heat.

Infections cause a unique response in the body. Bacteria, viruses, and other pathogens are identified as foreign invaders by our immune system. The immune system produces specific cells like white blood cells to eliminate these pathogens. A byproduct of this immunologic activity can sometimes be fever—a naturally occurring mechanism that raises body temperature in an effort to kill off pathogens.

Diseases impacting circulation like hypertension and atherosclerosis can alter the pathophysiology of various organs due to reduced blood flow. Hypertension puts extra strain on blood vessel walls, often leading to damage over time. Atherosclerosis involves plaque buildup within arteries which narrows them and thus restricts blood flow. As a result, organs may suffer from ischemia - inadequate blood supply - which can lead to tissue death if not addressed.

Additionally, chronic conditions such as diabetes impact various bodily functions. High levels of glucose in blood over time can damage nerves and small blood vessels, leading to complications like diabetic neuropathy—numbness or pain typically in feet or hands—and retinopathy which may impair vision.

Some vital concepts worth highlighting:

1. **Oxygen deprivation (hypoxia):** Cells require oxygen for metabolism; without it, they cannot function properly.

2. **Cell death (necrosis):** When cells die due to lack of nutrients or oxygen or due to toxins present from an infectious organism.

3. **Impaired function (dysfunction):** This occurs when organs do not operate normally as a result of disease or injury.

4. **Compensatory mechanisms:** These are body responses that attempt to maintain homeostasis despite challenges like fluid loss or changes in blood pressure.

Understanding these underlying physiological changes is critical for diagnostic purposes since they tend to manifest as symptoms we can observe and measure: pain from inflammation, coughing as a protective reflex from respiratory irritants, increased heart rate from shock or fever—you get the picture.

When assessing patients, EMTs must quickly identify symptoms that may signal underlying pathophysiological processes at work. For example, chest pain could indicate myocardial infarction caused by restricted blood flow to part of the heart muscle due to a blocked coronary artery.

Treatment decisions depend on identifying not just symptoms but understanding their pathophysiological causes—administering oxygen for hypoxia or administering certain medications that target specific dysfunctions. Recognizing and responding correctly can mean the difference between life and death or recovery versus long-term disability.

Pharmacology for EMTs

Pharmacology is the branch of medicine concerned with the uses, effects, and modes of action of drugs. It's important to understand how drugs interact with the human body. Once administered, a drug goes through four phases: *absorption, distribution, metabolism,* and *excretion* (ADME). Absorption concerns how a drug enters the bloodstream, which could be orally, intravenously, intramuscularly, sublingually, or through other routes. Distribution looks at how the drug disperses throughout the body. Metabolism involves the breakdown of the drug into active or inactive substances primarily by the liver. Lastly, excretion is how the drug or its metabolites exit the body usually via urine or feces.

Drugs can be categorized by their effects on the body or their therapeutic use. Some primary categories that EMTs should be familiar with include:

1. **Analgesics:** These are pain relievers and vary from over-the-counter medications like acetaminophen and ibuprofen to stronger opioid analgesics like morphine.

2. **Antiarrhythmics:** Used to treat heart rhythm disorders such as amiodarone or lidocaine.

3. **Anticonvulsants:** Help control seizures; examples include benzodiazepines like diazepam (Valium).

4. **Bronchodilators:** Alleviate respiratory issues by opening airways; commonly used ones include albuterol.

5. **Hypoglycemics:** Treat low blood sugar levels; oral glucose may be administered by EMTs.

6. **Narcotic antagonists:** Reverse effects of opioid overdose; naloxone (Narcan) is a common example.

7. **Vasoconstrictors:** Constrict blood vessels; one key example is epinephrine.

As an EMT, you'll need to understand the six *"rights"* of medication administration to ensure patient safety:

- Right patient
- Right medication
- Right dose
- Right route
- Right time
- Right documentation
- Routes of Administration

Medications can be administered in various ways. The route chosen depends on several factors including the drug's properties, desired speed of action, and patient condition.

1. **Oral:** Swallowed and absorbed through the stomach/intestinal lining.
2. **Sublingual:** Placed under the tongue for quick absorption into capillaries.
3. **Intramuscular (IM):** Injected into muscle tissue.
4. **Intravenous (IV):** Directly into a vein offering fastest delivery into bloodstream.
5. **Inhalation:** Breathed into the lungs often through nebulizers or inhalers.
6. **Transdermal:** Absorbed through layers of skin via patch formulations.
7. **Intraosseous (IO):** Injected directly into bone marrow when IV access cannot be established quickly; mostly used in critical care settings.

Determining correct dosages requires an understanding of medication concentration and patient-specific variables like weight and age. Always follow protocols and never exceed recommended dosages unless otherwise directed by medical control.

When assessing patients with potential for medication administration:

1. Check for allergies and ask about current medications to prevent adverse interactions.
2. Assess vital signs which could influence your choice of medication as well as its dosage.
3. If mental status is altered or competency is questionable, obtaining consent may involve speaking with next of kin when possible.

Lastly, as an EMT you are bound by both legal and ethical guidelines. You must have a clear understanding of your scope of practice and adhere to state laws governing EMTs. This includes not only when and how to administer medications but also how to obtain informed consent or operate under implied consent in an emergency. Always ensure that you are working within your certification level and do not attempt procedures or administer medications that exceed your training.

Documentation is a critical aspect of legality in pharmacology for EMTs. Properly recording all administered medications, dosages, routes, times, and the patient's response can protect you legally and improve patient care continuity. Remember, if it wasn't documented, it wasn't done.

It's also important to be aware of your local protocols which may vary by region and are often updated. Stay informed about changes and engage with continuous education opportunities.

CHAPTER 3
PATIENT ASSESSMENT FUNDAMENTALS

Scene Size-Up

In the vital phase of emergency medical services, conducting a proper scene size-up as the first step in patient assessment is paramount. This initial evaluation sets the stage for all subsequent actions and decisions made by emergency medical technicians (EMTs).

Scene size-up is the systematic approach taken by EMTs upon arrival at the scene of an emergency. It involves a quick yet comprehensive evaluation of the situation to ensure the safety of both EMS personnel and patients, determine the resources required, and identify potential hazards.

1. **Safety First:** Your safety comes first. On every call, quickly assess your safety, that of your team, and bystanders. Look out for signs of violence, disturbances, or environmental dangers. Be mindful of situational perils such as traffic on a highway or instability at a construction site.

2. **Nature of Call:** Establish what has happened. Gather information from dispatchers, updates en route, and observations upon arrival to surmise the nature and cause of the emergency. This will hint at potential risks and prepare you for patient contact.

3. **Personal Protective Equipment (PPE):** Before you dive into action, make sure you are protected from possible contaminants or bodily fluids that may transmit diseases. Gloves are essential, but depending on circumstances, you may also need masks, gowns, eye protection, or specialized equipment like HEPA respirators.

4. **Number of Patients:** Assess how many patients require medical attention as this determines additional EMS resources you might need to summon. Multiple patients can quickly escalate an incident's complexity and required response level.

5. **Additional Resources:** Does this situation require more hands or perhaps specialized units? If there are multiple patients or extrication is needed from damaged vehicles or precarious locations, backup is crucial—calling in police, fire services, or advanced medical support if necessary.

6. **Consider Spinal Precautions:** Early identification of potential spinal injury is critical as it influences how you approach patient care. Trauma from falls or motor vehicle accidents could warrant spinal immobilization protocols to prevent further injury.

7. **Scene Control:** Establish control by setting up boundaries and directing bystanders. Efficient management helps prevent additional injuries and maintains a safe working area for all responders.

8. **Environmental Factors:** Weather can largely impact patient assessment and care. Extreme conditions such as heat can exacerbate certain medical conditions while cold impacts your patient's body temperature and comfort level.

9. **Crowd Control:** A chaotic scene can be distracting and dangerous. Keep onlookers at bay to afford privacy to the patient and room for responders to work effectively.

10. **By-the-Book Communication:** Clear communication within your team and with other responding agencies ensures coordinated efforts; keep all parties informed about the developing situation and any changes in plans.

11. **Recognize Hazardous Materials Incidents:** If there is evidence of hazardous materials (Hazmat), keep a safe distance until Hazmat teams arrive. Your role here is to secure the perimeter until specialists can contain or neutralize hazards.

12. **Special Incident Management:** Certain situations such as mass injuries or casualties necessitate a disaster management approach including triage systems to prioritize care based on injury severity.

13. **Documenting Findings:** Document your scene size-up accurately as it's key information for ongoing care throughout EMS response.

Upon completing your thorough scene size-up at each call-out remember this fundamental principle remains steadfast - ensuring heightened vigilance toward safety cannot be understated in emphasizing its importance throughout patient assessment stages in prehospital care environments.

Remember also that patience is ongoing; scenes evolve rapidly therefore constant reassessment is paramount to adapting effectively whilst ensuring continuous protection for yourself and others involved.

Primary and Secondary Assessment

It is an intrinsic part of every EMS call and a foundational topic for NREMT (National Registry of Emergency Medical Technicians) study. The patient assessment process is methodically split into two crucial stages: the primary and secondary assessments.

The primary assessment, often termed the initial assessment, centers around rapidly identifying life-threatening conditions and addressing them immediately. This stage is succinctly encapsulated by the ABCDE mnemonic – *Airway, Breathing, Circulation, Disability,* and *Exposure/Environment.*

1. Airway assessment ensures that there is no obstruction preventing the patient from breathing. Seconds count here; if the airway is compromised, all ensuing efforts could be in vain. Without a patent airway, patients can quickly deteriorate and possibly result in death.

2. After confirming an open airway, rescuers assess whether the patient can adequately ventilate. This includes observing chest rise and fall, listening for breath sounds with a stethoscope, and checking skin color for indications of oxygenation.

3. Circulation investigates pulse quality, skin temperature, color, capillary refill time, and any signs of external bleeding. If circulation issues are detected or if there is major bleeding observable, these need immediate intervention to prevent shock or death.

4. Disability refers to assessing neurological status; this may include a quick evaluation using AVPU (Alert, Verbal response, Painful response, Unresponsive) scale or the Glasgow Coma Scale (GCS) in more detailed assessments.

5. Lastly, Exposure/Environment means removing clothing to inspect for injuries while simultaneously protecting patient privacy and preventing hypothermia.

These rapid steps must be completed within minutes because time can significantly affect outcomes. The primary goal is to detect and manage any life-threatening conditions before moving on to secondary assessment.

Once critical interventions are performed during the primary assessment or if no immediate threats are recognized, you move on to the secondary assessment. This extensive evaluation covers a complete head-to-toe examination and patient history taking.

The head-to-toe assessment starts at the cranial area checking for head injuries, then systematically moves down through all body parts until reaching extremities—inspecting for deformities, contusions, abrasions, punctures/penetrations, burns, tenderness, lacerations or swelling that could signify underlying injuries.

Simultaneously within this phase lies history-taking—a significant aspect involves using a tool called SAMPLE:

> ➢ S stands for Symptoms,
> ➢ A for Allergies,
> ➢ M for Medications,
> ➢ P for Past medical history,
> ➢ L for Last oral intake,
> ➢ E for Events leading up to the injury or illness.

Collecting this information may offer insights into possible medical complaints that aren't outwardly visible but can critically inform treatment decisions—such as allergic reactions complicating medical management or underlying health conditions influencing injury impacts.

Also integral in secondary assessment are vitals assessments—recording blood pressure readings; heart rate; respiratory rate; temperature; pulse oximetry for SpO2 levels; blood sugar levels where necessary; and pupils' examination for equality and reaction to light as they can indicate neurological issues.

First responders need this dual-assessment approach to prioritize immediate threats using primary evaluation then delve deeply into potential issues through secondary evaluation with systematic scrutiny including history gathering alongside vitals monitoring.

Vital Signs and Monitoring Devices

As a primary step in emergency patient assessment, understanding vital signs is crucial for aspiring EMTs. Vital signs offer a window into the physiological functions of the body, which can indicate the stability or distress of a patient's condition.

The pulse is a direct reflection of cardiac function and can reveal much about the heart's rhythm, strength, and speed. The normal pulse rate for an adult ranges from 60 to 100 beats per minute; however, this can vary due to factors such as age, fitness level, and even ambient temperature. When checking a pulse, you should also note the quality; whether it's strong or weak, regular or irregular. Common sites to palpate a pulse include the radial artery at the wrist and the carotid artery in the neck.

Next up is blood pressure – measured in millimeters of mercury (mmHg) – which comprises two readings: systolic and diastolic. Systolic refers to the pressure in arteries when the heart beats (the upper number), while diastolic represents pressure when the heart rests between beats (the lower number). A typical healthy reading is around 120/80 mmHg. Although automated devices can measure blood pressure, EMTs must also be proficient with a manual sphygmomanometer and stethoscope to avoid relying solely on electronic devices that may not always be available or accurate.

Respiratory rate, or the number of breaths per minute, is another key vital sign. For adults, 12–20 breaths per minute are considered normal. It is essential to observe not only the rate but also the quality of breathing – look for signs like gasping, wheezing, or labored breathing that could indicate respiratory distress. Maintaining a keen eye on chest movement can provide insights into potential thoracic injuries or obstructions.

Observing a patient's body temperature can tell you if they're feverish (typically above 100.4°F) or hypothermic (typically below 95°F), both of which could influence your treatment decisions. Oral thermometers are common for measuring temperature but in an emergency setting where trauma is involved or when patients are unresponsive, alternative methods like tympanic (ear) or temporal artery thermometers might be used.

Oxygen saturation is often considered an additional vital sign; this measures how much oxygen your blood carries compared to its full capacity. Measured using a pulse oximeter clipped to a finger tip, normal levels range from 95% to 100%. Numbers below this range could indicate hypoxia - insufficient oxygen reaching tissues.

Monitoring devices such as pulse oximeters have become standard EMT equipment due to their portability and ease of use. These small devices provide real-time readings of oxygen saturation as well as pulse rate – allowing for quick assessments even in transit.

Another crucial piece of equipment is the automated external defibrillator (AED). While not used for regular assessments, AEDs are vital to have at hand during cardiac emergencies as they diagnose life-threatening arrhythmic conditions of the heart such as ventricular fibrillation and pulseless ventricular tachycardia and treat them through defibrillation. Understanding how to operate an AED properly is mandatory for every EMT.

Documentation plays an essential role in patient assessment as accurate records ensure continuity in care once handed over to emergency department personnel. Details of all vital signs taken should be noted down correctly along with observations made during assessments using monitoring equipment and monitored over time. This includes any abnormalities or changes in the patient's condition that may indicate a decline or improvement. Accurate record-keeping can greatly impact the efficacy of the hand-off process and, ultimately, patient prognosis.

A thorough understanding and competent assessment of vital signs are indispensable tools in the EMT's repertoire. By mastering these skills, EMTs can better triage patients, prioritize care based on severity, and make informed decisions about treatment and transport. It is essential to remember that vital signs should not be viewed in isolation but rather as part of a comprehensive patient assessment that includes medical history, chief complaint, and physical examination.

CHAPTER 4
AIRWAY MANAGEMENT

Airway Anatomy and Physiology

Airway anatomy is a complex structure, meticulously designed to provide two essential functions: respiration and protection. The airway begins at the nose and mouth, where air is inhaled, passing through the pharynx and down into the larynx—commonly known as the voice box. Herein lies the epiglottis, a leaf-shaped flap, which serves as a switchboard directing food to the esophagus and air to the trachea.

The trachea sits below the larynx and acts as a conduit sending air into the lungs. Lined with cilia and mucous membranes, it also plays a role in filtering out particulate matter. This 'windpipe' then bifurcates into two primary bronchi—one for each lung—before subdividing into smaller bronchioles capped by millions of alveoli, tiny sacs where gas exchange takes place.

Let's delve deeper into physiology—the science of how these anatomical structures function during respiration. Breathing begins with ventilation, moving air in (inspiration) and out (expiration) of your lungs. During inspiration, muscles like the diaphragm and intercostal muscles contract, creating negative pressure that allows air to flow into your lungs. Expiration is usually passive; these muscles relax, pushing air out of your lungs.

Oxygen from inhaled air diffuses across alveolar walls into pulmonary capillaries, binding to hemoglobin in red blood cells—a process essential for cellular metabolism and energy production throughout your body. Meanwhile, carbon dioxide, a byproduct of metabolism, diffuses from blood to alveoli to be exhaled.

Now comes inherent challenges that EMTs must navigate—the threat of airway obstruction. An unobstructive pathway is crucial for effective breathing but can be compromised by several factors such as swelling from allergic reactions or anaphylaxis, foreign objects like food or small toys in children, or bodily fluids from trauma patients.

Recognizing signs of an obstructive airway is pivotal for swift EMT intervention. Signs include abnormal breathing sounds such as stridor or wheezing, use of accessory muscles for breathing, cyanosis around lips or fingertips pointing towards hypoxia—a state of insufficient oxygen reaching tissues—and altered level of consciousness indicating immediate danger.

Airway Management

Airway clearance techniques are crucial skills for any emergency medical technician (EMT) or healthcare professional responding to respiratory emergencies. They are procedures used to aid in the removal of mucus and other secretions from the airways, which help maintain open air passages, ensuring effective ventilation and oxygenation of the patient.

One common technique is coughing and deep breathing exercises. These exercises encourage the patient to take deep breaths and cough forcefully to mobilize secretions. As an EMT, you can assist patients by guiding them through these exercises—asking them to take a deep breath, hold it for a second, and then cough sharply. This can be especially helpful after an incident that might lead to atelectasis or during transport of patients with chronic lung diseases.

Chest physiotherapy (CPT) is another method used to help clear the airways. This involves clapping the patient's chest and back with cupped hands to loosen mucus so it can be coughed up more easily. The technique requires training, as improper force or frequency could cause discomfort or injury. CPT is often used in conjunction with postural drainage, where a patient is positioned in a way that uses gravity to assist in draining secretion from different lobes of the lungs.

Mechanical devices such as percussion vests or handheld devices may also be employed for airway clearance. Percussion vests vibrate at high frequencies against the chest to loosen mucus and secretions in the lungs. Handheld devices like flutter valves create pressure and vibrations when a patient exhales through them, helping move mucus toward the larger airways where it can be coughed out.

Endotracheal suctioning is used when a patient is unable to clear secretions on their own due to altered consciousness or when there's an artificial airway in place like an endotracheal tube. As an EMT, you must meticulously adhere to sterile technique during suctioning to prevent introducing infections into the lower airways.

Oxygen therapy is also essential for patients struggling with airway clearance; it provides supplemental oxygen to aid in maintaining adequate tissue oxygenation when natural airway-clearing mechanisms fail. As part of your patient assessment, checking pulse oximetry will help determine the necessity of oxygen supplementation in conjunction with clearance techniques.

Lastly, medication nebulizers can assist with airway clearance by delivering drugs that thin secretions (mucolytics) or dilate bronchial passages (bronchodilators). During your care for patients with conditions such as asthma or chronic obstructive pulmonary disease (COPD), nebulizer treatments may be administered pre-transport if approved by medical direction protocols.

As EMTs responding to calls involving respiratory distress or failure, you must be proficient in these techniques and understand when each is appropriate. Always follow local protocols and consult medical control as necessary for guidance on performing advanced techniques.

Ventilation Devices and Oxygen Delivery

Ventilation devices and oxygen delivery are essential components in emergency medical care, especially for patients who are experiencing respiratory distress or failure. Understanding these devices is crucial for effective respiratory support and can be lifesaving.

Ventilation devices come in various forms, each designed for specific situations and patient needs. One common device is the **Bag-Valve Mask (BVM)**, often used in pre-hospital settings. The BVM consists of a self-inflating bag, a one-way valve, and a face mask. It allows first responders to deliver breaths manually to a patient who is not breathing adequately or at all. Proper sealing of the mask on the patient's face is important to ensure efficient delivery of oxygen while minimizing air leakage.

Another important device is the **Pocket Mask**, which has a one-way valve and is connected to an oxygen inlet. It is smaller than a BVM and facilitates mouth-to-mask ventilation. The rescuer breathes through the one-way valve, which filters out exhaled air, delivering oxygen from an attached source directly to the patient.

Automatic Transport Ventilators (ATVs) are sophisticated devices providing consistent ventilation to patients during transport. They're programmed to deliver a set volume or pressure of air per breath at a specific rate and are used when high-quality manual ventilation is difficult to maintain over time.

Oxygen delivery systems aim to increase the amount of oxygen inhaled by patients who aren't getting enough naturally. The simplest form is the **Nasal Cannula**, which delivers low levels of supplemental oxygen. It consists of a flexible tube with two small prongs that fit just inside the nose. This system allows for mobility and comfort while helping patients with less severe breathing problems.

Simple Face Masks cover both the nose and mouth of patients and connect to an oxygen source to deliver higher amounts of oxygen than nasal cannulas. These masks have exhalation ports allowing carbon dioxide to escape.

Non-Rebreather Masks include a reservoir bag that stores pure oxygen from the connected supply, allowing higher concentrations of oxygen delivery (upward of 90%). Exhalation valves prevent the exhaled air from entering the reservoir, meaning only pure oxygen from the bag is inspired. They are used in more critical cases where high levels of supplemental oxygen are required.

Venturi Masks deliver precise concentrations of oxygen by mixing room air with pure oxygen and are particularly useful when consistent and specific levels of supplemental oxygen need to be maintained.

In advanced airway management, **Endotracheal Tubes (ETs)** provide an open passage through the trachea directly to the lungs allowing for mechanical ventilation with precise control over breathing patterns and protection from aspiration. ETs require substantial training as the placement involves intubation — inserting the tube into a patient's windpipe.

Laryngeal Mask Airways (LMAs) offer an alternative method for securing an airway without intubation into the trachea; instead, they sit above the glottis within the pharynx providing another means for ventilatory support during emergencies.

It is crucial for NREMT candidates to understand not just how these devices work but also their appropriate use based on patient assessment — evaluating breathing rate, depth, effort, lung sounds, skin color, and mental status. Also instrumental in decision-making is understanding indications and contraindications — knowing when it's safe and beneficial versus potentially harmful to use each device.

Efficient use of these devices also includes recognizing and managing potential complications that might arise. For example, while using a BVM, inadequate seal or excessive ventilation force can lead to gastric insufflation, where air is pushed into the stomach instead of the lungs, potentially causing vomiting and aspiration. Similarly, when using nasal cannulas or masks, it's critical to monitor for signs of skin breakdown or discomfort, particularly around the ears or bridge of the nose.

High-flow oxygen therapy is a newer development in oxygen delivery that is increasingly being used in emergency settings. High-flow nasal cannula (HFNC) systems can deliver warmed and humidified oxygen at much higher flows than standard devices, improving patient comfort and oxygenation. This method allows for better control of the fraction of inspired oxygen (FiO2) and provides a level of positive airway pressure which can aid in keeping airways open.

Capnography is another tool often used alongside ventilation devices to monitor the concentration of carbon dioxide in exhaled air, reflecting the adequacy of ventilation. This non-invasive monitoring can be critical in ensuring proper function of devices and alerting providers to respiratory issues before they become life-threatening.

Continuous training and simulation practice are imperative for proficiency with these tools. Moreover, guidelines from bodies like the American Heart Association are regularly updated, so practitioners must stay informed about best practices.

CHAPTER 5
CARDIOLOGY AND RESUSCITATION

Cardiovascular Emergencies

Cardiovascular emergencies are critical conditions that affect the heart and blood vessels and require immediate medical attention. These emergencies can be life-threatening and often need urgent intervention to restore blood flow, treat underlying causes, and support the affected individual's cardiovascular system.

One of the most common cardiovascular emergencies is a **heart attack**, or **myocardial infarction**. This occurs when the blood flow to a part of the heart is blocked, usually by a blood clot. Without timely treatment, the affected heart muscle begins to die due to a lack of oxygen-rich blood. Signs and symptoms of a heart attack can include chest pain or discomfort that may radiate to the back, neck, jaw, or arms, shortness of breath, sweating, and nausea.

Another serious condition is **cardiac arrest**, where the heart suddenly stops beating properly, interrupting blood flow to the brain and other vital organs. Cardiac arrest can result from various causes, including a heart attack, drowning, an electrical shock, or severe trauma. A person experiencing cardiac arrest will be unresponsive and won't have a detectable pulse.

In cases of suspected cardiac arrest, *immediate cardiopulmonary resuscitation (CPR)* can be life-saving. CPR involves chest compressions combined with rescue breathing to manually circulate blood and provide oxygen to the body's organs until professional medical help arrives or normal heart rhythm is restored with an automated external defibrillator (AED).

Chest compressions should be performed at a rate of 100–120 per minute and at a depth of about 2 inches (5 cm) on an adult patient. The rescuer should allow for complete chest recoil between compressions and minimize interruptions during CPR. If available and trained for use, an AED can be used after 5 cycles of CPR or approximately two minutes if no return of spontaneous circulation (ROSC) is achieved.

Congestive Heart Failure (CHF) is another common cardiovascular emergency that requires prompt recognition and treatment. CHF occurs when the heart does not pump effectively enough to meet the body's needs. Fluid can build up in the lungs and other tissues leading to difficulty breathing, swelling in legs and ankles, fatigue, irregular heartbeat, and persistent coughing or wheezing.

Emergency treatment for CHF may involve positioning the patient upright to ease breathing discomfort if they are conscious; providing oxygen therapy if saturation levels are low; monitoring vital signs closely; administering nitroglycerin if prescribed; and rapid transport for hospital evaluation.

Hypertensive emergencies are severe elevations in blood pressure that could result in acute organ damage such as hypertensive encephalopathy, stroke, or acute myocardial infarction. Signs include severe headache, nosebleed, altered mental status or confusion accompanied by extremely high blood pressure readings.

Patients in hypertensive emergency may require intravenous medications to lower their blood pressure gradually in a controlled setting as rapid reduction may lead to ischemia or organ damage.

In any cardiovascular emergency situation—it's essential for first responders to remain calm while quickly assessing the scene's safety before aiding the patient; they must also work efficiently in team-coordinated efforts if multiple responders are present.

Keep in mind that all these interventions pending arrival at an emergency department are intended as immediate measures meant to sustain life as every second counts during cardiovascular events affecting someone's heart rhythm and function.

Automated External Defibrillation

Automated External Defibrillators (AEDs) have become a critical component in the chain of survival for patients experiencing sudden cardiac arrest (SCA). As pre-hospital emergency care providers, understanding the function and operation of AEDs is essential. The design of most AEDs is user-friendly, allowing even untrained bystanders to use them effectively with prompt guidance.

Sudden cardiac arrest occurs when the heart's electrical system malfunctions, typically resulting in an arrhythmia called ventricular fibrillation (VF) or ventricular tachycardia (VT) without a pulse. In these situations, immediate defibrillation can be life-saving. An AED is a portable device that checks the heart rhythm and can send an electric shock to the heart to try to restore a normal rhythm.

Quick response times are crucial when dealing with SCA. The chances of survival decrease by 7-10% with each passing minute without defibrillation. Hence, it is imperative for bystanders and first responders to initiate immediate resuscitation efforts including the use of an AED.

When using an AED, it's important to follow a step-by-step process:

1. **Ensure Safety:** Before using an AED on a patient, make sure that the surrounding area is safe for both the patient and the rescuer. Remove the patient from water if necessary and look out for any potential hazards.

2. **Turn on the AED:** As soon as you retrieve it, turn on the AED; it will provide voice-activated instructions which should be followed precisely.

3. **Expose Patient's Chest:** Open or remove clothing to expose the patient's chest completely. If there's a lot of hair where the pads should go, quickly shave the area if possible with razors typically provided with an AED kit.

4. **Attach Pads:** Apply sticky pads equipped with sensors (electrodes) directly to the patient's bare chest as indicated by pictures on the pads.

5. **Clear Patient:** Ensure no one is touching or bumping into the patient or bed during analysis and prior to shock delivery.

6. **Analyze Heart Rhythm:** Allow the AED to analyze the heart rhythm; don't touch the patient during this time as movement may disrupt reading.

7. **Deliver Shock if Necessary:** If directed by the device, ensure all individuals are standing clear of contact with patient and press the 'shock' button once ready.

8. **Initiate CPR After Shock:** Immediately after delivering a shock, begin CPR starting with chest compressions unless otherwise instructed by emergency personnel or if the patient starts showing signs of life like coughing or moving spontaneously.

It's vital that all steps are followed swiftly and calmly to give patients the highest chance of survival until advanced life support personnel can take over.

In addition to understanding how to operate an AED, recognizing that these devices have algorithms specifically designed for either adult or pediatric patients (usually less than eight years old or weighing less than 55 pounds) is important. Pediatric pads and/or settings must be used for children since they deliver a reduced-energy shock appropriate for smaller hearts; however, if only adult pads are available they may be used as a last resort following specific placement instructions for children.

The presence of implantable devices like pacemakers or defibrillators among patients should also be noted by rescuers who are using an AED. Pads should not be placed directly over these devices as it might interfere with their operation. Instead, place one pad in the center of the chest between nipples and another on the back between shoulder blades if this situation arises.

Time and efficiency are everything in cardiac emergencies. The sooner an AED is applied and a shock delivered if necessary, the better the outcome for the patient. To maximize effectiveness, AEDs should be included in regular emergency drills and training sessions for both public spaces and professional responders.

Post-resuscitation care after AED use is equally important to patients' survival. Once the patient's heart rhythm is restored and they begin to show signs of life, they must receive comprehensive medical evaluation and care to address any underlying conditions and prevent potential recurrence of cardiac arrest.

Ensuring widespread public access to AEDs can improve survival rates. This involves placing AEDs in high-traffic areas such as airports, schools, gyms, and shopping malls. Public awareness campaigns about the importance and simplicity of using AEDs can encourage more people to act during a cardiac emergency.

CPR for Adults, Children, and Infants

Cardiopulmonary resuscitation (CPR) is a life-saving technique useful in many emergencies, including heart attack or near drowning, where someone's breathing or heartbeat has stopped. It's critical for saving lives and improving chances of survival. CPR for adults, children, and infants differ slightly in technique, reflecting the differences in anatomy and physiology.

For adults, the process begins by verifying that the person is unresponsive and not breathing normally. Once confirmed, call 911 and begin chest compressions. Place the heel of one hand on the center of the person's chest, with your other hand on top, interlocking your fingers while keeping your arms straight. Press down hard and fast at least 2 inches deep but not exceeding 2.4 inches at a rate of 100 to 120 compressions per minute. After every 30 compressions, give two rescue breaths by tilting the head back to open the airway, lifting their chin, pinching their nose shut, and making a complete seal over their mouth with yours before blowing in to make the chest clearly rise.

When it comes to children between one year old and puberty, CPR starts similarly by ensuring they're unresponsive and not breathing normally. Call for emergency medical services or instruct someone else to do so if you're alone with the child, continue with CPR. The compression technique is similar but uses less force; compress about 2 inches deep at the same rate as for adults. Rescue breaths are also required after every 30 compressions but be gentle as children's lungs are smaller; do not blow as hard as you would for an adult.

For infants under one year old, things change slightly because they are more delicate and their structures are smaller. If you find an infant unresponsive and not breathing normally after you've tried waking them up gently, call for help or direct someone else to call. Perform CPR by placing two fingers at the center of the infant's chest just below the nipple line. Compress about 1.5 inches deep at a rate of 100 to 120 compressions per minute. After every 30 compressions, perform two rescue breaths by making a complete seal over both their nose and mouth with your mouth and breathe gently into their lungs to achieve a visible rise in their chest.

In all cases of CPR for adults, children, or infants:

➤ Ensure that you provide high-quality chest compressions by pushing hard and fast in the center of the chest.

- ➢ Allow complete recoil after each compression.
- ➢ Minimize interruptions in compressions.
- ➢ Avoid excessive ventilation; only give enough air during rescue breaths to make the chest visibly rise.

Time is critical when administering CPR; effective bystander CPR provided immediately after sudden cardiac arrest can double or triple a victim's chance of survival. Remember that even if you're unsure about your ability to perform CPR correctly, it's better to attempt resuscitation than do nothing at all. Good Samaritan laws protect those who act in good faith trying to save a life.

CHAPTER 6
MEDICAL AND OBSTETRICS/ GYNECOLOGY

Medical Assessment Strategies

Start with the primary survey; this includes assessing the patient's Airway, Breathing, and Circulation (ABC). Make sure the airway is open and clear. If not, take immediate action to rectify it. Then, check their breathing—is it regular, paced, or erratic? Finally, examine their circulation. Are their pulses strong and uniform? Once ABCs are secure, reassess them frequently throughout your care.

Next is capturing an accurate history. Use SAMPLE as your mnemonic: Symptoms, Allergies, Medications, Past medical history, Last oral intake, and Events leading up to the illness or injury. A thorough history can often give clues to the underlying issues at hand.

Vital signs are next. A patient's temperature, blood pressure, pulse rate, respiratory rate, and oxygen saturation can all indicate what's going wrong inside their body. Get a baseline for comparison later on.

The secondary assessment involves a systematic physical examination from head to toe for trauma patients or focused where necessary for medical patients. Check all areas while maintaining respect for patient comfort and privacy. Lastly, regularly reassess your patient to monitor for any changes in their condition. This may influence your decisions on further management or transport necessities.

Managing Common Medical Emergencies

With medical emergencies ranging from chest pain to diabetic crises to seizures, there's an array of conditions that an EMT might encounter.

For chest pain suggestive of a heart attack (acute coronary syndrome), time is muscle. Provide oxygen if hypoxic, reassurance to ease anxiety and prepare for rapid transport. If protocols allow and the patient has no contraindications—like a known allergy or blood pressure too low—administer aspirin which can help prevent further clot formation in the coronary arteries.

Asthma attacks are another frequent encounter whereby individuals may experience difficulty in breathing due to inflamed airways. Positioning them upright helps breathing while providing supplemental oxygen if needed. Administer prescribed inhalers or nebulized treatments if you have them available as they open constricted airways.

For diabetic emergencies such as hypoglycemia where a patient might exhibit confusion or unconsciousness due to low blood sugar levels—the administration of oral glucose can be lifesaving if they're awake enough to swallow; otherwise intravenous dextrose may be required.

Seizures demand immediate attention—ensure that the patient is safe from injury during convulsions but do not restrain them or put anything in their mouth. Afterward place them in the recovery position to maintain an open airway and continue monitoring vital signs.

Another common yet life-threatening event you might face is stroke; here early identification is key as certain types—specifically an ischemic stroke—can be treated with medications that dissolve clots if given within a specific time frame after symptom onset. Look out for facial droop, arm weakness or speech difficulties (FAST) as indicators and expedite transport.

Obstetrical Emergencies and Childbirth

Obstetrical emergencies are acute medical situations that occur during pregnancy, labor, or immediately after delivery. These emergencies can pose a significant risk to the mother, fetus, or both. An understanding of these conditions is essential for pre-hospital care providers, including those preparing for the National Registry Emergency Medical Technician (NREMT) examination.

1. **Ectopic Pregnancy:** This occurs when a fertilized egg implants outside the uterus, often in a fallopian tube. Recognizing ectopic pregnancy is crucial because if the tube ruptures, it can lead to life-threatening bleeding. Signs include abdominal pain on one side, vaginal bleeding, and dizziness.

2. **Preeclampsia:** A condition characterized by high blood pressure and protein in the urine after the 20th week of pregnancy. Symptoms may include severe headaches, visual disturbances, upper abdominal pain, and swelling of the hands and feet. If left untreated, it can lead to seizures (eclampsia) or stroke.

3. **Placenta Previa:** The placenta covers all or part of the cervix inside the uterus. It can cause severe bleeding before or during delivery. Key signs are painless vaginal bleeding in the second half of pregnancy.

4. **Placental Abruption:** The separation of the placenta from the uterine lining before delivery. It can cause severe abdominal pain and vaginal bleeding. This is an emergency situation because it can compromise fetal oxygen supply.

5. **Umbilical Cord Prolapse:** This occurs when the umbilical cord slips into the vagina before or during delivery. Prompt recognition is critical since it can result in fetal suffocation if unnoticed. Signs include a sudden decrease in fetal heart rate and visible cord in the vagina after membrane rupture.

6. **Amniotic Fluid Embolism:** An unpredictable condition where amniotic fluid enters the mother's bloodstream causing cardiovascular collapse. It presents with sudden respiratory distress, hypotension, seizures, and coagulopathy. Immediate advanced life support measures are required.

7. **Postpartum Hemorrhage (PPH):** Excessive bleeding following childbirth. PPH is defined as a loss of more than 500 ml of blood after vaginal delivery or 1000 ml after cesarean section. Causes include uterine atony, retained placental fragments, lacerations, and coagulopathy.

Childbirth involves three phases—the first stage (dilation), second stage (expulsion), and third stage (delivery of the placenta). In a normal vaginal delivery process:

1. **Dilation Stage:** Begins with regular contractions leading to cervical dilation up to 10 cm.
2. **Expulsion Stage:** Active pushing and delivery of the baby.
3. **Placenta Stage:** Delivery of the placenta typically occurs within 5–30 minutes after birth.

During childbirth:

➢ Encourage effective pushing only during contractions to optimize maternal efforts.
➢ Monitor fetal heart rate; normally ranges between 120 to 160 beats per minute.
➢ Ensure there is no prolapse of umbilical cord.

After birth:

➢ Rub newborn's back or gently stimulate to encourage crying which expands their lungs.
➢ Clamp and cut umbilical cord following medical protocols.
➢ Deliver placenta while avoiding excessive pulling on cord which may cause uterine inversion.
➢ Control any maternal bleeding.

For all obstetrical emergencies:

➢ Provide high-flow oxygen as needed for mother.
➢ Initiate IV access with large bore needles for potential fluid/blood replacement.
➢ Monitor vital signs frequently.
➢ Transport patient on left side if possible to avoid supine hypotensive syndrome where gravid uterus compresses inferior vena cava reducing blood return to heart.

The management of obstetrical emergencies requires swift action and expertise. To ensure the best possible outcomes, pre-hospital care providers must be equipped with a specific set of skills and knowledge.

CHAPTER 7
TRAUMA EMERGENCIES

Trauma Assessment and Management

Traumatic injuries can occur from a wide variety of incidents, such as motor vehicle collisions, falls, assaults, and accidents at home or in the workplace. The initial assessment of a trauma patient is paramount to their survival. Prior to rendering aid, ensure that the environment around both you and the patient is secure. Once safety is established, proceed with your primary assessment.

Begin with the ABCDEs – Airway, Breathing, Circulation, Disability (neurological status), and Exposure/Environmental control.

1. **Airway** – Open the airway using a jaw-thrust maneuver if you suspect spinal injuries or a head-tilt-chin-lift if you do not. Check for obstructions such as blood, vomit, or foreign objects.
2. **Breathing** – Assess the patient's breathing. Look for chest rise and fall, listen for breath sounds, and feel for breath on your cheek. Administer high flow oxygen or assist ventilations with a bag-valve mask (BVM) if necessary.
3. **Circulation** – Check for major bleeding; control it with direct pressure or tourniquets if life-threatening. Feel for a pulse to determine circulation status and perfusion quality.
4. **Disability** – Assess the patient's level of consciousness using the AVPU scale which stands for Alert, Verbal response, Painful stimulation response, Unresponsive. Also check pupils for size and reactivity.

5. **Exposure/Environmental control** – Remove clothing to assess for injuries but ensure you maintain the patient's privacy and warmth.

After addressing immediate life threats during your primary survey, move on to a secondary survey if time and patient condition permit. In this detailed head-to-toe assessment, look for additional signs of injury and gather a patient history following the SAMPLE acronym: Symptoms, Allergies, Medications currently used, Past relevant medical history/injuries/surgeries/etc., Last oral intake (food/drink), Events leading up to the injury or illness.

During your assessment and management of trauma patients:

1. Be thorough in your examination but prioritize interventions that address immediate life threats.
2. Reassess regularly to identify changes in condition.
3. Take C-spine precautions with any trauma patient due to potential neck/back injuries until cleared by appropriate imaging/diagnostics.
4. Consider internal bleeding as an underlying cause of shock in cases with no obvious external blood loss.
5. Anticipate complications such as tension pneumothorax or cardiac tamponade in blunt chest trauma.
6. Time is tissue — make swift decisions based on rapid assessments.

Document findings promptly and accurately; information you gather during these initial stages can be critical for subsequent caregivers in the emergency department or hospital setting.

Effective trauma management involves not only addressing physical injuries but also providing emotional support. Stay calm and reassure your patient throughout your encounter—your demeanor can influence their physiological response to injury.

Remember that behind every task performed lies the goal of preserving life, preventing further injury, and promoting recovery. As an EMS professional studying for NREMT certification or recertification, knowing these principles is crucial because when it comes to trauma emergencies every second counts.

It is important to note that protocols may vary slightly by region or country; however, these guidelines offer a fundamental approach to trauma emergencies suitable for NREMT study purposes. Proper training coupled with hands-on experience will deepen your understanding beyond this study guide's foundation —for mastery lies in the practice of these essential lifesaving skills.

Bleeding and Shock

Uncontrolled bleeding is a life-threatening condition that can lead to shock, a state of inadequate tissue perfusion and oxygenation. When approaching a trauma scene, ensuring Scene Safety is paramount before assessing the patient. Once safe, identify the source of bleeding.

Bleeding can be external or internal. External bleeding is often visible, exhibiting as bright red spurts in arterial bleeding or dark oozing in venous bleeding. Internal bleeding is more insidious but may present with signs such as tachycardia, hypotension, distended abdomen, or bloody urine or stool.

The initial step in managing bleeding is to apply direct pressure with a clean dressing. If this fails to control the bleed and if appropriate training is held, consider hemostatic agents or tourniquets as next levels of intervention. Remember to reassess the effectiveness of these interventions continually.

Shock occurs when the vascular system fails to provide sufficient blood circulation to body tissues and vital organs. The primary types of shock relevant in trauma are hypovolemic (due to fluid loss), cardiogenic (due to heart failure), obstructive (due to blockage of blood flow), and distributive (due typically to severe infection or spinal cord injury).

Recognition signs include pale skin, cool to touch, rapid pulse rate but weak in nature, low blood pressure, altered mental status, and delayed capillary refill time (CRT). Immediate treatment involves maintaining airway patency, providing high-concentration oxygen if available and indicated by oxygen saturation levels and patient condition.

Positioning the patient plays a role in shock management; typically placing them in a supine position benefits most shock states by facilitating perfusion. Additionally, preserving body warmth helps prevent temperature-related augmentation of shock state.

Soft Tissue and Musculoskeletal Injuries

Soft tissue injuries include contusions, abrasions, lacerations, avulsions, punctures, burns and blast injuries can result from blunt force or penetrating trauma. Controlling infection risk and promoting healing are primary goals in the treatment process.

Cleanse abrasions with mild soap solutions as long as there are no underlying fractures suspected. For deeper wounds like lacerations or avulsions ensure bleeding control first before covering with a sterile dressing.

Burns require special attention depending on their depth; superficial burns involve only the top layer of skin while partial thickness burns create blisters; full thickness burns char skin deeply affecting multiple layers including potentially muscles and bones beneath them — manage pain appropriately using non-entangling dressings while avoiding popular misconceptions such as applying ice directly onto burns which can worsen tissue damage further.

Musculoskeletal injuries range from sprains/strains up through complex fractures/ dislocations which destabilize anatomical structures causing pain along with potential compromises in circulation dependent on severity/location relative each injury's specific characteristics.

When assessing musculoskeletal trauma look for Deformities Contusions Abrasions Punctures/Eviscerations Burns Tenderness Lacerations Swelling — 'DCAP-BTLS', a mnemonic useful for remembering these indicators.

Splinting immobilizes injured extremities to prevent further damage while awaiting definitive care. To splint effectively, you must immobilize the joint above and below the injury. Use splints that are rigid, well-padded, and long enough to stabilize the injury. However, if you suspect a spinal injury, spinal precautions must be taken.

In cases of suspected fractures or dislocations, check circulation, sensation, and motor function in the injured limb before and after splinting. If there's a vascular compromise or severe neurologic injury, Emergency Medical Services (EMS) personnel should expedite transport and provide continuous monitoring en route to the hospital.

Traction splints are specifically designed for femur fractures and can alleviate pain, prevent further damage to soft tissues, and reduce blood loss. These should only be applied by individuals with appropriate training as improper use can exacerbate the injury.

For dislocations, it is imperative not to attempt to reposition or reduce the joint in the field. Maintain stabilizing support for the joint in its current position with a splint or sling until definitive care can be provided at a medical facility.

CHAPTER 8
INFANTS AND CHILDREN

Pediatric Assessment and Care

When it comes to pediatric patients, infants and children bring their own set of challenges to the table. Accurate assessment and appropriate care for these young patients are essential for anyone preparing for the NREMT examination.

Infants, defined as those under one year of age, and children, who range from one year to adolescence, possess physiological differences that can affect not only their presentation during an emergency but also your approach to treatment. Their airway structures are smaller and more easily obstructed, they have faster metabolic rates requiring different considerations when dealing with fluid and medication dosages, and they may not be able to communicate what is wrong or how they feel.

In the initial assessment of an infant or child, focus on life-threatening issues first by using the Pediatric Assessment Triangle (PAT), which includes evaluating appearance (tone, interactiveness, consolability, look/gaze, speech/cry), work of breathing (abnormal breath sounds, positioning), and circulation to the skin (pallor, cyanosis). Remember that in pediatric assessment, parental involvement is necessary not only for information purposes but also to help comfort the child.

For infants especially, use a gentle but methodical approach. Observe them in their parent's arms first rather than immediately separating them, which could lead to unnecessary stress and crying that complicates your assessment. When you do handle infants for detailed physical examinations or procedures such as measuring vital signs or administering medication or oxygen, explain your actions calmly to the parent(s) and perform your actions swiftly but gently.

Vital signs in children vary with age and must be evaluated against pediatric specific norms. Tachycardia or bradycardia can be serious signs of distress or illness. Respirations should be observed without disturbing the child if possible since agitated breathing might not give an accurate reflection of their normal state. Temperature regulation is also different in infants and children – they're more susceptible to heat loss due to a larger surface area–to–volume ratio yet might not manifest fever as readily due to less effective heat generation capacities.

For respiratory emergencies in children such as asthma or bronchiolitis, your key interventions include ensuring airway patency and providing oxygen therapy while considering smaller dosage needs for medications like albuterol. In cardiac situations like congenital heart defects presenting in infancy or arrhythmias in older children, recognizing signs early on during assessment can be lifesaving.

When assessing circulation check pulses carefully—they may be more difficult to locate on small limbs—and keep in mind that signs of shock may appear late due to children's compensatory mechanisms. If circulation is compromised you may need fluid resuscitation tailored not just in volume but also considering different fluid types appropriate for younger systems.

Trauma requires a proportionately larger emphasis on spinal precautions due to the greater head-to-body ratio in infants and small children. When immobilizing a pediatric patient for transport, be particularly attentive not simply for anatomical reasons but also emotional consideration; offering reassurance throughout the process is key.

Common Pediatric Emergencies

Pediatric emergencies often present a unique set of challenges for emergency medical services (EMS) professionals. When assessing and treating infants and children, it's crucial to understand the common medical emergencies they may face. Some of the most prevalent emergencies include respiratory distress, seizures, fever, dehydration, and trauma.

Respiratory distress can manifest in various ways, such as grunting, wheezing, or stridor. Children have smaller airways than adults, so obstructions can be particularly dangerous for them. Asthma is a common chronic condition that may lead to acute exacerbations requiring immediate medical attention. EMS providers should be prepared to administer oxygen therapy and potentially assist in ventilation if necessary.

Seizures in children may be related to fevers (febrile seizures) or other neurological conditions like epilepsy. During a seizure, it's essential to protect the child from injury and to maintain their airway open once the seizure has stopped. Postictal care is also important, as children often require comfort and reassurance along with a thorough assessment to determine the cause of the seizure.

Fever is another frequent pediatric emergency; while it's typically a sign of infection, in young children even relatively minor infections can precipitate serious conditions such as sepsis. It's important for EMS personnel to assess for other signs of serious illness when a child presents with a fever.

Dehydration may occur due to vomiting, diarrhea, or insufficient fluid intake. In infants and young children, dehydration can escalate quickly and become life-threatening. Signs of dehydration include dry mucous membranes, decreased tear production, sunken eyes, and in severe cases, delayed capillary refill time. Resuscitation with fluids can be a critical intervention.

Trauma in children requires careful evaluation because their responses to injury may differ from adults. Due to their size and anatomical differences, children are more susceptible to certain types of injuries such as those involving the head and abdomen. The assessment must also consider non-accidental trauma (child abuse), which may necessitate additional legal and social interventions besides medical care.

Special Considerations for Infants and Children

When providing emergency care for infants and children, there are special considerations that should be kept in mind by all EMS providers:

1. **Airway management:** As mentioned earlier, the airway of a child is smaller than an adult's. Furthermore, their airway anatomy is proportionally different – for example, infants have larger heads compared to their bodies which influences their airway

position. Providers must be trained in pediatric-specific airway management techniques including positioning and equipment selection.

2. **Developmental differences:** Recognizing that children are not just small adults is key; their bodies respond differently physiologically to illness and injury. For instance, they have faster heart rates but can quickly decompensate once they exhaust their compensatory mechanisms.

3. **Communication:** Infants cannot verbalize their needs while older children may be frightened or uncooperative during medical emergencies. Techniques for calming children include using gentle tones, explaining procedures using simple language they can understand (when appropriate), allowing them to hold onto a favorite toy or blanket when possible, and engaging them visually.

4. **Dosages:** Medications dosages must always be calculated based on weight rather than standardized adult dosages; using pediatric-specific medication dosage aids like Broselow tapes can help reduce errors.

5. **Equipment sizes:** All equipment used must correspond accurately to the child's size – from endotracheal tubes to blood pressure cuffs – since using equipment that's too large or too small can result in injury or inaccurate readings.

6. **Family involvement:** Family members are crucial both as sources of information about the child's medical history and current symptoms, and for comforting the child during assessment and treatment. Involving a parent or guardian in the care process can help ease a child's anxiety. However, it should be balanced with the need to perform medical interventions promptly and efficiently.

7. **Legal considerations:** Consent for treatment in the pediatric population is often provided by a parent or guardian, but there are circumstances where consent is implied, such as when a child is in critical condition and a legal guardian is not present. EMS providers should be familiar with laws concerning treatment of minors in emergency situations.

CHAPTER 9
OPERATIONS

Principles of EMS Operations

The operations within EMS revolve around a set of core principles designed to ensure that patient care is timely, efficient, and coordinated. At the heart lies the commitment to save lives and alleviate suffering, which drives every decision made on the job. From preparation to execution, these principles are pivotal.

One such principle is preparedness. Preparedness embodies the training, equipment maintenance, and continued education necessary for emergency medical technicians (EMTs) and paramedics to remain at peak readiness. Every call demands that personnel be equipped with not only medical knowledge but also an understanding of the devices and tools they carry in their ambulances.

Communication is next in line but equal in importance. From the initial 911 call to handover at the hospital, clear communication ensures everyone involved — dispatchers, first responders, law enforcement, fire services, and medical staff — knows their roles and ongoing situational details.

Safety extends beyond patient care to encompass providers as well. Ensuring a scene is safe for EMS personnel upon arrival is essential. They are trained to observe their surroundings for potential hazards — chemical spills or unstable structures, for example — before providing patient care.

Quality improvement is an ongoing process within EMS operations that involves reviewing calls after completion to identify successes and areas needing improvement. Continuous learning from past experiences helps elevate the level of care provided.

Patient advocacy means acting in the best interest of patients who may not always be able to make crucial decisions due to their medical condition or stress levels during an emergency. It requires emotional intelligence beyond clinical expertise – understanding when to reassure a frightened victim or obtaining consent from relatives when necessary.

Incident Management and Multiple-Casualty Incidents

In the event of an emergency that involves multiple casualties, effective incident management becomes the cornerstone of a successful response. At the heart of this management system is the Incident Command System (ICS), a standardized approach to the command, control, and coordination of emergency response. The ICS allows agencies and personnel from different departments to work together towards a common goal, creating an organized response to incidents that may otherwise be chaotic.

Multiple-Casualty Incidents are situations where the number of victims exceeds the immediately available resources. These incidents require careful triage, which is the process of prioritizing patients based on the severity of their conditions. Following established triage protocols, such as START (Simple Triage and Rapid Treatment), helps ensure that those in most need receive immediate attention.

During an MCI, establishing a command post is crucial for effective management. The command post serves as a centralized point for leadership and decision-making. Personnel roles are divided into different sectors, including operations, logistics, planning, finance/administration, and safety. Communication among all sectors and with other responding agencies is vital.

EMS plays a pivotal part in MCIs by providing medical evaluation, care, and transportation to hospitals with appropriate resources to handle the influx of patients. Scene safety is emphasized throughout operations to ensure that EMS personnel can perform their duties without additional risks.

Ground and Air Ambulance Operations

Ground ambulances are often the primary mode of transport in an emergency medical situation, used for transferring patients from the scene to a medical facility or between facilities. The function of ground ambulance operations includes ensuring vehicles are well-maintained, properly equipped, and staffed with trained EMTs ready to deliver pre-hospital care.

The interior of a ground ambulance is designed to act as a mobile emergency treatment center equipped with essential lifesaving equipment such as oxygen delivery systems, defibrillators, backboards, splinting devices, bandages, medication administration kits like auto-injectors for allergic reactions or IV supplies for fluid replacement, sphygmomanometers (blood pressure cuffs), stethoscopes, patient monitoring devices, and communication equipment.

Safety in ground ambulance operations extends beyond patient care during transport; it also incorporates safe driving practices adhering to traffic laws while also taking into consideration factors like weather conditions or road types which could affect response times or patient comfort during transport.

Air ambulances come into play when rapid transport is crucial due to distance or when terrain makes ground travel impractical or impossible – situations often seen in rural or wilderness settings. Helicopters typically used as air ambulances have similar medical equipment on board compared to ground ambulances but usually have advanced capabilities like ventilators due to longer transport times.

Flight paramedics and nurses on air ambulances must have specialized training not only in advanced medical procedures but also in understanding aviation principles since they must factor in altitude physiology and aircraft safety principles when caring for patients mid-flight.

Whether through ground or air transport methods involving strict adherence to protocols ensures fast yet secure passenger delivery crucial during what may be life-altering moments for those being served by EMTs nationwide.

CHAPTER 10
ADVANCED PREPARATION TECHNIQUES

Study Strategies for the NREMT

The NREMT is designed to test not only your knowledge but also your ability to apply it in various scenarios. To prepare effectively, consider implementing the following strategies:

1. **Active Learning:** Simply reading textbooks or attending lectures is often insufficient. Engage in active learning by teaching the material to others, discussing concepts with peers, or applying what you've learned through practical exercises or simulations.

2. **Practice Tests:** One of the most valuable tools in your arsenal should be practice exams. Not only do they familiarize you with the format and style of questions you'll encounter, but they also identify areas where you may need additional study.

3. **Daily Review Sessions:** Short, frequent study sessions help reinforce learning better than marathon cramming sessions. Dedicate at least 30 minutes each day to review material you've covered previously.

4. **Organized Study Groups:** Collaborative learning can be powerful if structured properly. Join or form a study group with dedicated and disciplined individuals who are as committed as you are to passing the NREMT.

5. **Time Management:** Balance your study schedule with breaks to avoid burnout—your brain needs time to absorb information and recover from intense study sessions.

Memory aids are invaluable tools for recalling vast amounts of information. Here are some techniques tailored for memorizing medical procedures and terminology:

1. **Mnemonics:** Create simple, catchy acronyms or phrases to remember sequences or lists—like "SAMPLE" for collecting a patient history (Symptoms, Allergies, Medications, Past medical history, Last oral intake, Events leading up).
2. **Visualization:** Harness the power of visual memory by creating mental images or diagrams that link together pieces of information in a memorable way.
3. **Storytelling:** Turn complex concepts into narratives or stories where each element represents a part of the information you need to remember.
4. **Chunking:** Break down long strings of information into smaller, manageable chunks that are easier to memorize—one example is segmenting a drug dosage calculation into parts rather than trying to remember it as a whole.

Time Management and Study Plans

Effective time management is vital when preparing for any exam—especially one as intensive as the NREMT.

1. **Set Realistic Goals:** Establish clear, achievable goals for each study session to keep focused and motivated throughout your preparation journey.
2. **Create a Schedule:** Dedicate specific times of day for studying, break sessions into manageable chunks, and stick to your schedule religiously to ensure consistent progress.
3. **Prioritize Topics:** Since certain areas of the exam carry more weight than others, prioritize your studies accordingly, allocating more time to high-yield content without neglecting less prevalent topics.
4. **Regular Review:** Incorporate regular review sessions into your plan to reinforce learning over time and avoid cramming before the exam date.
5. **Self-Care Breaks:** Include short breaks for rest throughout your schedule; mental fatigue can lead to diminished retention, so it's important to unwind periodically.
6. **Accountability:** Partner with a study group or find an accountability buddy who can help you stay on track with your plan while offering support and encouragement along the way.

47

CHAPTER 11
NREMT PRACTICE TESTS AND EXPLANATIONS

Full-Length Practice Test: Medical Emergencies

1. Which of the following is NOT a sign of myocardial infarction (MI)?

   A. Chest pain radiating to the left arm
   B. Sudden dizziness and sweating
   C. A rapid, fluttering heartbeat
   D. Increased blood pressure

2. What is the first line treatment for a patient exhibiting signs of congestive heart failure (CHF)?

   A. Immediate tracheal intubation
   B. Nitroglycerin administration
   C. High flow oxygen therapy
   D. Intravenous fluid bolus

3. A patient is presenting with an irregular pulse, chest discomfort, and confusion. The ECG shows chaotic and irregular waves with no discernible P waves or QRS complexes. What is the most appropriate course of action?

    A. Synchronized cardioversion

    B. Defibrillation

    C. Administration of intravenous atropine

    D. Immediate start of CPR

4. When treating a patient with suspected acute coronary syndrome (ACS), which medication would you administer cautiously?

    A. Aspirin

    B. Nitroglycerin

    C. Atropine

    D. Epinephrine

5. For a patient experiencing a hypertensive emergency with a sudden onset of severe headache and nosebleed, which is the most immediate concern?

    A. Referral to a cardiologist

    B. Monitoring neurological status

    C. Lowering blood pressure gradually

    D. Nasal packing to stop nosebleed

6. Which rhythm will you typically find on the ECG of a patient suffering from Torsades de Pointes?

    A. Sinus bradycardia

    B. Wide complex tachycardia with 'twisting' QRS complexes

    C. Regular narrow complex tachycardia

    D. Asystole

7. For a patient with suspected acute myocardial infarction (AMI), which medication should be administered first provided there are no contraindications?

    A. Oral glucose.

    B. Nitroglycerin sublingually.

    C. Aspirin chewable tablets.

    D. Morphine intravenously.

8. Which rhythm should you be prepared to defibrillate?

    A. Sinus bradycardia

    B. Ventricular fibrillation (VF)

    C. First-degree AV block

    D. Sinus rhythm with PACs

9. Which of the following is a common sign of a tension pneumothorax?

    A. Tracheal deviation away from the affected side

    B. Slow, deep respirations

    C. Bilateral wheezing

    D. Unilaterally equal breath sounds

10. A patient experiencing an acute asthma attack is likely to present with:

    A. Prolonged expiration and wheezing

    B. Rapid improvement with mild exertion

    C. Decreased level of consciousness as an early sign

    D. Stridor on inhalation

11. What is an indication for CPAP in respiratory distress?

    A. Decreased blood pressure

    B. Frothy sputum at the mouth and nose

    C. Gurgling respirations

    D. Respiratory arrest

12. In cases of suspected pulmonary embolism, what is the most appropriate initial action?

    A. Administer a thrombolytic immediately.

    B. Apply oxygen and transport promptly.

    C. Perform endotracheal intubation.

    D. Start chest compressions.

13. For a patient with flail chest, you may notice:

    A. Paradoxical movement of the chest wall section.

    B. Hyperresonance upon chest percussion.

    C. A barrel-shaped chest upon inspection.

    D. Decreased respiratory rate to reduce pain.

14. You arrive on scene to find a patient presenting with audible wheezes, use of accessory muscles, tripod positioning, and speaking in incomplete sentences. The primary cause is most likely:

A. Asthma exacerbation

B. Myocardial infarction

C. Croup

D. Hyperventilation syndrome

15. The presence of jugular venous distension (JVD), muffled heart sounds, and hypotension in a trauma patient strongly suggests:

A. Tension pneumothorax

B. Cardiac tamponade

C. Acute myocardial infarction

D. Congestive heart failure

16. When assessing a patient with suspected hyperventilation syndrome, which of the following would be least likely to be observed?

A. Carpopedal spasm

B. Tachycardia

C. Pinpoint pupils

D. Numbness in the extremities

17. Which of the following is a common sign of a stroke?

A. Muscle atrophy

B. High fever

C. Slurred speech

D. Photophobia

18. A patient presents with sudden-onset severe headache, photophobia, and neck stiffness. What is the most likely diagnosis?

A. Tension headache

B. Migraine

C. Subarachnoid hemorrhage

D. Temporal arteritis

19. When assessing a patient with a suspected traumatic brain injury, what is the priority?

    A. Checking for pupil reactivity

    B. Assessing the level of consciousness

    C. Checking blood glucose levels

    D. Immediate intubation

20. Which of the following actions should be taken first for a patient experiencing a generalized tonic-clonic seizure?

    A. Restrain the patient to prevent injury

    B. Insert an oral airway

    C. Position the patient to ensure an open airway and await cessation of seizure activity

    D. Administer oral glucose

21. In cases of suspected bacterial meningitis, which intervention should be initiated after airway, breathing, and circulation have been assessed?

    A. Immediate antibiotics administration

    B. Administration of diuretics

    C. Cold compresses to forehead

    D. Elevating the foot end of the bed

22. What focal neurological deficit is commonly seen with an epidural hematoma?

    A. Bilateral weakness in legs

    B. Sudden blindness

    C. Hemiparesis on one side of the body

    D. Loss of proprioception

23. You arrive at a scene where a patient appears confused and combative after a motor vehicle collision, these symptoms may indicate:

    A. Normal post-accident stress reaction

    B. Intracerebral hemorrhage

    C. Alcohol intoxication

    D. Hypoglycemia

24. A 68-year-old female with history of hypertension suddenly cannot move her right arm and leg when waking up this morning. She is likely suffering from:

   A. Peripheral neuropathy
   B. Ischemic stroke
   C. Bell's palsy
   D. Multiple sclerosis flare-up

25. Which of the following signs and symptoms would MOST likely suggest an abdominal aortic aneurysm?

   A. Sudden onset of flank pain with radiation to the shoulder
   B. Gradual onset of epigastric pain with vomiting
   C. Tearing pain with a pulsating abdominal mass
   D. Consistent pain in the lower abdomen with rebound tenderness

26. A 45-year-old male complains of sudden onset of severe, sharp epigastric pain radiating to the back. He admits to heavy alcohol use. What is the MOST likely diagnosis?

   A. Acute pancreatitis
   B. Peptic ulcer disease
   C. Cholecystitis
   D. Appendicitis

27. Which condition is characterized by sudden onset of pain in the right lower quadrant, fever, and rebound tenderness?

   A. Diverticulitis
   B. Cholecystitis
   C. Appendicitis
   D. Ulcerative colitis

28. During your assessment of a patient with suspected gastrointestinal bleeding, you notice that the patient has melena. What does this indicate?

   A. Bright red blood in vomit indicating active upper GI bleed
   B. Bright red blood per rectum indicating lower GI bleed
   C. Black, tarry stools indicating a bleed somewhere in the upper GI tract
   D. Grey, clay-like stools indicating gallbladder disease

29. You are assessing a patient who presents with severe epigastric pain and appears pale and anxious. His vital signs show tachycardia and hypotension. What emergency condition should you suspect?

    A. Gastroesophageal reflux disease (GERD)
    B. Perforated peptic ulcer
    C. Esophageal varices
    D. Irritable bowel syndrome (IBS)

30. For a patient presenting with upper abdominal discomfort that is relieved by eating food or taking antacids but returns several hours after eating is most indicative of what condition?

    A. Gastritis
    B. Esophageal varices
    C. Peptic ulcer disease
    D. Pancreatitis

31. In cases of suspected acute cholecystitis, which symptom is MOST characteristically reported by patients?

    A. Pain in the right shoulder after eating
    B. Pain in the left lower quadrant associated with fever
    C. Sudden, intense pain in the upper right quadrant that may radiate to the back
    D. Gradual abdominal swelling with associated nausea

32. A patient presents with severe dehydration, hypotension, and a history of vomiting and diarrhea for the past 48 hours. Which electrolyte imbalance should be a concern?

    A. Hypercalcemia
    B. Hypokalemia
    C. Hypernatremia
    D. Hypermagnesemia

33. What is the primary physiologic problem in Type 1 diabetes mellitus?

    A. Insulin resistance
    B. Overproduction of insulin
    C. Absence of insulin production
    D. Hyperactivity of glucagon hormone

34. What is a common early sign of hyperglycemic hyperosmolar syndrome (HHS)?

    A. Hypotension
    B. Polydipsia
    C. Bradycardia
    D. Muscle weakness

35. An EMT finds a diabetic patient unresponsive with cold, clammy skin. What should be the first step in management?

    A. Oral glucose administration
    B. Rapid IV fluid replacement
    C. Checking blood glucose level
    D. Cardioversion

36. Which one of these actions can precipitate diabetic ketoacidosis (DKA)?

    A. Skipping meals after taking insulin
    B. Consuming high sugar food items
    C. Overexercising without nutritional compensation
    D. Intense stress or infection

37. Which electrolyte imbalance is most critical to address in a patient with severe diabetic ketoacidosis?

    A. Hyponatremia
    B. Hypercalcemia
    C. Hypokalemia
    D. Hyperphosphatemia

38. During an assessment of a potential endocrine emergency, which symptom would suggest thyroid storm over hypothyroidism?

    A. Weight gain and lethargy
    B. Cold intolerance and depression
    C. Fever and tachycardia
    D. Constipation and bradycardia

39. The administration of what medication is most appropriate for a conscious patient experiencing hypoglycemia with the ability to swallow?

    A. Intravenous dextrose 50%

    B. Glucagon injection

    C. Oral glucose gel/tablet

    D. Aspirin

40. Which of the following is a potential consequence of untreated hypoglycemia in diabetic patients?

    A. Diabetic coma

    B. Metabolic alkalosis

    C. Euthyroid sick syndrome

    D. Parathyroid gland hypertrophy

41. Which of the following signs or symptoms is most indicative of an allergic reaction?

    A. Localized itching

    B. Abdominal pain

    C. Peripheral edema

    D. Hives and itching

42. What is the primary treatment for anaphylaxis in the prehospital setting?

    A. High-flow oxygen

    B. Oral antihistamines

    C. Intramuscular epinephrine

    D. Intravenous corticosteroids

43.You arrive on scene to find a patient who was stung by a bee and is now having difficulty breathing. You note swelling around the neck area. What should you suspect?

    A. A stroke

    B. Anaphylaxis

    C. Asthma attack

    D. Angioedema

44. Which patient would be at greatest risk for developing anaphylaxis?

   A. A diabetic patient with a skin infection.
   B. A patient with known allergies who was just exposed to their allergen.
   C. A patient with hypertension taking beta-blockers.
   D. A child with no known allergies.

45. One of the early signs of an allergic reaction that can precede anaphylaxis is:

   A. Slurred speech.
   B. A sense of impending doom.
   C. Coughing.
   D. Profound tachycardia.

46. When treating a patient experiencing an acute allergic reaction, it is important to:

   A. Place the patient supine and elevate their legs.
   B. Administer high-concentration oxygen if respiratory distress or hypoxia is present.
   C. Provide reassurance and avoid any medications due to possible reactions.
   D. Elicit a complete medication history before any treatment.

47. The "Five Rights" are important when administrating epinephrine for anaphylaxis. These include all EXCEPT:

   A. Right time
   B. Right route
   C. Right documentation
   D. Right expiration date

48. When assessing a patient with suspected anaphylaxis, what should you check first?

   A. Capillary refill
   B. Airway patency
   C. Blood pressure
   D. Skin condition

49. Which substance abuse is MOST likely to result in depressive symptoms upon withdrawal?

   A. Cocaine
   B. Alcohol
   C. Heroin
   D. Methamphetamine

50. What is the antidote for acetaminophen overdose?

    A. Flumazenil
    B. Naloxone
    C. Activated charcoal
    D. Acetylcysteine

51. During an opioid overdose, what clinical sign is MOST indicative of this type of poisoning?

    A. Hyperthermia
    B. Constricted pupils (miosis)
    C. Agitation
    D. Hypertension

52. Which of the following drugs is classified as a stimulant?

    A. Diazepam
    B. Amphetamine
    C. Hydrocodone
    D. Marijuana

53. A patient suspected of ingesting a large quantity of benzodiazepines should be monitored for what primary complication?

    A. Seizures
    B. Respiratory depression
    C. Hallucinations
    D. Hyperactivity

54. What defines "tolerance" in the context of substance abuse?

    A. The capability to stop using a substance at will without difficulty.
    B. The need for increasing substance amounts to achieve the same effect.
    C. A reduced response upon repeated exposure to the same amount of a substance.
    D. Experiencing withdrawal symptoms when a substance is discontinued.

55. In which situation would activated charcoal NOT be recommended for an overdose patient?

    A. Overdose on aspirin taken one hour ago.
    B. Overdose on lithium taken two hours ago.
    C. Patient ingested corrosive substances.
    D. Patient overdosed on ibuprofen three hours ago.

56. Which medication is an appropriate treatment for benzodiazepine overdose?

    A. Flumazenil

    B. Naloxone

    C. Acetylcysteine

    D. Atropine

57. What is the most appropriate immediate care for a patient with heat stroke?

    A. Move the patient to a cooler environment and apply cool packs to the groin, armpits, and neck.

    B. Provide the patient with small sips of water if conscious.

    C. Wrap the patient in warm blankets to gradually lower body temperature.

    D. Encourage physical activity to aid the cooling process through sweat.

58. Which of the following breathing difficulties should be expected in a patient suffering from anaphylaxis after a bee sting?

    A. Slow, deep respirations

    B. Wheezing on inspiration and expiration

    C. Rapid, shallow respirations

    D. No difficulty in breathing

59. What is the first step in treating a patient with suspected frostbite to their fingers?

    A. Vigorously rub the affected area to generate heat.

    B. Immediately immerse the fingers in hot water.

    C. Remove any wet clothing and provide gentle rewarming of the affected area.

    D. Break any blisters that have formed to release fluid pressure.

60. When treating a snake bite, why is it important not to apply ice to the affected area?

    A. Ice can increase venom absorption into surrounding tissues.

    B. Cold temperatures are soothing and may slow down medical care.

    C. Applying ice can reduce swelling caused by the bite.

    D. The snake's venom may react with ice, causing a chemical burn.

61. How should you assist a responsive patient with mild hypothermia who is shivering vigorously?

    A. Have them perform intense exercise.

    B. Get them into dry clothing and wrap them in blankets.

    C. Place them in a hot bath to quickly raise body temperature.

    D. Offer them alcoholic beverages to help them feel warm.

62. In case of a carbon monoxide poisoning emergency, what is your initial step as an emergency responder?

    A. Administer high-flow oxygen via nonrebreather mask if available.

    B. Ask patients about recent headaches or flu-like symptoms for diagnosis confirmation.

    C. Start chest compressions if the patient has no pulse.

    D. Perform abdominal thrusts if they are vomiting.

63. What is the best treatment for a patient experiencing the "bends" (decompression sickness)?

    A. Immediate administration of aspirin for pain relief.

    B. 100% oxygen and prompt recompression therapy.

    C. Drinking plenty of fluids to stay hydrated.

    D. Encouragement to walk around to improve circulation.

64. During a lightning storm, how can you increase a patient's safety if they are outdoors and unable to find shelter?

    A. Lie flat on the ground to reduce your profile.

    B. Seek shelter under tall trees for protection.

    C. Find a low-lying area away from water, trees, and metal objects, and assume a crouched position with only the feet touching the ground.

    D. Keep walking to different locations hoping to avoid potential lightning strikes.

65. Which of the following infectious diseases is transmitted primarily through airborne droplets?

    A. Hepatitis B

    B. Human Immunodeficiency Virus (HIV)

    C. Tuberculosis (TB)

    D. Methicillin-resistant Staphylococcus aureus (MRSA)

66. What is a common sign or symptom of severe sepsis?

    A. Hypertension

    B. Warm, dry skin

    C. Decreased urine output

    D. Patient reporting a feeling of wellness

67. Which hepatitis virus is most commonly transmitted through contaminated food and water?

    A. Hepatitis A

    B. Hepatitis B

    C. Hepatitis C

    D. Hepatitis D

68. What protection should EMS providers use when treating a patient with suspected meningococcal meningitis?

    A. Gloves only

    B. Gloves and face shield

    C. Gloves, gown, and N95 mask

    D. Gloves, gown, face shield, and N95 mask

69. A patient presents with fever, headache, and a stiff neck. These symptoms are most indicative of which condition?

    A. Influenza

    B. Meningitis

    C. Hepatitis B

    D. Mononucleosis

70. HIV can be contracted through which of the following body fluids?

    A. Sweat

    B. Tears

    C. Saliva

    D. Semen

71. After initial influenza infection, symptoms typically develop within what time frame?

    A. 1 to 4 hours

    B. 12 to 36 hours

    C. 1 to 4 days

    D. 5 to 7 days

72. Early recognition and treatment are critical for patients with suspected Ebola virus disease because:

    A. The mortality rate remains high despite medical care.

    B. Antibiotics need to be administered as early as possible.

    C. It can prevent the disease from spreading within the community.

    D. All of these reasons are correct.

73. When first approaching a patient with signs of a psychiatric emergency, what is the most important initial action?

    A. Restrain the patient immediately for their safety.

    B. Establish a therapeutic rapport and ensure the scene is safe.

    C. Begin immediate transportation.

    D. Perform a rapid physical assessment.

74. Which of the following is an effective de-escalation technique when managing patients with behavioral emergencies?

    A. Invading the patient's personal space to show authority.

    B. Using closed-ended questions that can be answered with 'yes' or 'no.'

    C. Speaking loudly and quickly to show urgency.

    D. Maintaining calm demeanor and using active listening skills.

75. Which medication is commonly used for chemical restraint in an agitated patient during psychiatric emergencies?

    A. Metformin

    B. Haloperidol

    C. Albuterol

    D. Furosemide

76. When transporting a potentially violent psychiatric patient, what precautionary measure should be taken?

    A. Leave the patient unrestrained so as not to escalate anxiety or agitation.

    B. Keep talking to the patient constantly to divert their attention.

    C. Place restraints as deemed necessary while ensuring proper circulation and respiratory function.

    D. Have one crew member sit in the back of the ambulance with the patient at all times without any escape route.

77. What is an important question to ask during evaluation of a suicidal patient in the pre-hospital setting?

    A. "Why do you feel life isn't worth living?"

    B. "Do you have an elaborate plan for how you would commit suicide?"

    C. "Can any staff members here persuade you otherwise about your feelings?"

    D. "Have others treated you unfairly, leading you to this point?"

78. Substance abuse can often exacerbate or cause which of these behavioral emergencies?

    A. Orthostatic hypotension

    B. Hypoglycemia

    C. Panic attacks

    D. Seizures

79. During a psychiatric emergency, how can bystanders be most helpful?

    A. By crowding around the patient to observe.

    B. Restraining the patient until help arrives.

    C. Offering the patient food or drink to calm them down.

    D. Giving the responding emergency personnel space to work and following their instructions.

80. What must EMS providers maintain regarding a patient's personal health information during a psychiatric emergency?

    A. Divulge information to law enforcement regardless of necessity.

    B. Share details with bystanders who are curious about the situation.

    C. Maintain confidentiality according to HIPAA regulations.

    D. Discuss patient information freely once off-duty.

81. Which of the following signs is NOT commonly associated with preeclampsia?

    A. Hypertension
    B. Proteinuria
    C. Hyporeflexia
    D. Edema

82. First-line treatment for a mother suffering from postpartum hemorrhage immediately after delivery should include:

    A. Supine positioning with leg elevation
    B. Application of a tourniquet to the lower extremities
    C. Immediate administration of oral fluids
    D. Massaging the uterus while checking for retained placental parts

83. Which symptom is MOST indicative of a possible ectopic pregnancy in a patient experiencing abdominal pain?

    A. Intermittent nausea and vomiting
    B. Vaginal bleeding with a positive pregnancy test
    C. A history of amenorrhea followed by lower abdominal cramping
    D. Acute onset diarrhea without fever

84. The recommended immediate management action when encountering prolapsed umbilical cord during delivery is:

    A. Apply gentle traction on the cord to relieve pressure
    B. Encourage the mother to push harder to expedite delivery
    C. Position the mother with her hips higher than her head or in knee-chest position and provide high-flow oxygen
    D. Clamp and cut the umbilical cord immediately

85. Which of the following is an essential component of managing gestational diabetes?

    A. Administering regular insulin injections, regardless of blood glucose levels
    B. Performing daily aerobic exercise without obstetrician approval
    C. Monitoring maternal blood glucose levels and maintaining a balanced diet
    D. Restricting fluid intake to prevent fetal overgrowth

86. What is the MOST urgent concern when treating a patient with suspected ovarian torsion?

    A. Immediate administration of pain medication

    B. Surgical intervention to correct the torsion

    C. Frequent pelvic examinations to assess changes

    D. Application of heat to the lower abdomen to relieve discomfort

87. Which symptom is MOST characteristic of placenta previa in the second or third trimester?

    A. Sudden, painless vaginal bleeding

    B. Abdominal pain and tender uterus on palpation

    C. Sudden onset of rhythmic contractions

    D. Excessive vomiting with dehydration

88. What is the FIRST step in managing shoulder dystocia during delivery?

    A. Delivering the posterior arm first

    B. Performing an immediate Caesarean section

    C. Applying suprapubic pressure while encouraging maternal pushing

    D. Using fundal pressure to dislodge the anterior shoulder

Full-Length Practice Test: Trauma Emergencies

89. When dealing with a patient who has sustained significant soft tissue trauma to the forearm with profuse bleeding, what is the first and most appropriate step to control the bleeding?

    A. Apply a tourniquet immediately above the injury site.

    B. Elevate the limb above heart level.

    C. Apply direct pressure with a clean cloth or dressing.

    D. Administer high-flow oxygen.

90. In managing an open chest wound that is suspected to be a tension pneumothorax, what is the most suitable procedure?

    A. Perform needle decompression.

    B. Cover the wound with a flutter-valve dressing.

    C. Apply direct pressure to stop bleeding.

    D. Deliver rescue breaths at a higher rate.

91. What sign can indicate internal bleeding in a trauma patient?

    A. Rapid, strong pulse.

    B. Cold and clammy skin.

    C. Localized pain to injury site.

    D. Bright red blood spewing from an injury site.

92. With regard to soft tissue injuries, what does the term 'ecchymosis' refer?

    A. A jagged laceration.

    B. Swelling due to fluid accumulation in tissue spaces.

    C. The blue or purplish discoloration of the skin due to leaked blood vessels.

    D. An avulsion where skin is torn from the body.

93. When treating a patient with an amputated finger, how should you preserve the amputated part for potential reattachment?

    A. Wash it with water, wrap it in sterile gauze, and keep it on ice.

    B. Place it directly on ice.

    C. Keep it warm by placing it next to the patient's body.

    D. Wrap it in dry sterile gauze and place it in a plastic bag kept cool with ice.

94. Which of these scenarios is an indication for applying a tourniquet?

    A. A deep cut on the scalp with moderate bleeding controlled by direct pressure.

    B. A puncture wound on the torso with minimal external bleeding.

    C. An extremity injury with profuse bleeding not controlled by direct pressure or dressings.

    D. Any open wound which continues to bleed after being elevated above heart level.

95. Which condition is considered a life-threatening complication of severe soft tissue trauma and should be monitored for in all trauma patients?

    A. Compartment syndrome.

    B. Tachycardia.

    C. Fractures.

    D. Hypothermia.

96. What is the recommended treatment for a chemical burn to the skin after ensuring the scene is safe?

    A. Apply an oil-based ointment to soothe the skin.

    B. Flush the affected area with large amounts of water.

    C. Immediately neutralize the chemical with an acid or alkali.

    D. Cover the burn with dry dressings and avoid cooling measures.

97. Which of the following should be the first step in the pre-hospital care of a burn patient?

    A. Apply cool, damp cloths

    B. Check for airway patency

    C. Administer high-flow oxygen

    D. Cover the burn with sterile dressings

98. A patient with full-thickness burns on their hands should be treated by:

    A. Applying ice packs to the burned areas.

    B. Immersing the hands in cold water.

    C. Elevating the hands and covering them with a dry, sterile dressing.

    D. Rubbing antibiotic ointment on the burns.

99. When assessing a burn's severity, which factor is considered?

    A. Patients' age and preexisting medical condition

    B. The size of the person's hand used to estimate TBSA

    C. Color of burnt area only

    D. Location of the burn on the body

100. What is the most appropriate way to estimate the total body surface area (TBSA) affected by a burn?

    A. Rule of Nines

    B. Patient's palm method

    C. Lund and Browder chart

    D. Both A and C are correct

101. Which type of burn usually requires surgical intervention due to its depth?

    A. Superficial burn

    B. Partial-thickness burn

    C. Full-thickness burn

    D. All burns require surgical intervention

102. In managing chemical burns, what is an important initial step?

    A. Assess for bone fractures.

    B. Snap pictures for medical records.

    C. Remove contaminated clothing carefully.

    D. Apply a tourniquet above the wound.

103. For a patient suffering from inhalation injury due to a burn, what symptom would you expect to find upon assessment?

    A. Slurred speech

    B. Peripheral edema

    C. Singed nasal hairs or sooty sputum

    D. Increased thirst

104. What is a unique concern when treating electrical burns?

    A. They always require amputation.

    B. They are not painful so they can be ignored.

    C. The extent of injury may be greater internally than it appears externally.

    D. Application of liberal amounts of ointments

105. When treating a patient with a suspected femur fracture, which of the following is the most appropriate initial action?

    A. Immobilize the leg with a traction splint.

    B. Apply a cold pack to the injured area.

    C. Administer high-flow oxygen.

    D. Assess distal pulse, motor, and sensory function.

106. What is the key sign to differentiate between a dislocation and a fracture?

    A. Presence of bruising

    B. Severe pain

    C. Deformity at the site of injury

    D. Loss of distal pulses

107. You arrive on scene to find a patient who fell off a ladder complaining of severe wrist pain. How should you manage this patient's injury?

    A. Check for radial pulse before any further assessment.

    B. Splint the wrist in the position found.

    C. Have the patient move their fingers to assess for fractures.

    D. Attempt to realign any deformities observed.

108. During your assessment of a car accident victim, you note that her foot is pointing laterally instead of forward. Considering possible musculoskeletal trauma, your first intervention should be:

    A. Quickly realign her foot to its natural position.

    B. Begin immediate transport without interventions.

    C. Check for neurovascular integrity before other interventions.

    D. Stabilize her foot as is and prepare for transport.

109. What type of musculoskeletal injury involves an over-stretching or tearing of ligaments around a joint?

    A. Fracture

    B. Dislocation

    C. Sprain

    D. Strain

110. In a case of suspected ankle sprain, what is the most appropriate initial treatment?

    A. Apply heat to the affected area to increase blood flow.

    B. Encourage the patient to walk it off as it may just be stiffness.

    C. Use the R.I.C.E method - Rest, Ice, Compression, Elevation.

    D. Provide high-flow oxygen and transport.

111. What is the most reliable method to confirm a diagnosis of fracture?

    A. Palpation of the injury site for tenderness.

    B. Visual assessment for deformity.

    C. X-ray imaging of the affected area.

    D. Checking for neurovascular impairment.

112. Which of the following signs is MOST indicative of increased intracranial pressure?

    A. Constricted pupils

    B. Hypertension

    C. Bradycardia

    D. An irregular respiratory pattern

113. In a case of suspected spinal injury, which of the following actions is most appropriate when managing the patient's airway?

    A. Head-tilt chin-lift maneuver

    B. Jaw-thrust maneuver without head extension

    C. Aggressive suctioning of the airway

    D. Hyperextension of the neck for better airway alignment

114. You arrive on scene to find an unconscious patient from a fall with a clear fluid draining from their nose. You suspect this fluid to be cerebrospinal fluid. This finding is often associated with:

    A. A basilar skull fracture

    B. Nasal bone fracture

    C. Sinusitis

    D. Allergic rhinitis

115. A football player was hit from behind and is complaining of numbness in his legs. Initial assessment reveals no open injuries but there is deformity to his cervical spine area. What is your immediate action?

A. Apply high-flow oxygen via non-rebreather mask.

B. Immobilize his spine manually until further assessments can be made.

C. Transfer him onto a stretcher without delay.

D. Perform a detailed neurologic exam on the field.

116. During the secondary assessment of a patient with head trauma, you notice bruising around the patient's eyes and behind the ears. These signs are characteristic of:

A. A concussion

B. A hematoma

C. A basilar skull fracture

D. Orbital fractures

117. When assessing a patient with a suspected spinal injury, it is important to check for:

A. Priapism

B. Hyperreflexia in the extremities

C. Tension headache

D. Slurred speech

118. What is the most appropriate method to assess motor function in a patient with suspected cervical spine injury?

A. Ask the patient to shrug their shoulders.

B. Ask the patient to move their hands and fingers.

C. Have the patient perform deep knee bends.

D. Instruct the patient to walk and observe their gait.

119. A patient has sustained blunt trauma to the eye. Which of the following signs should MOST concern the EMT?

A. The patient is experiencing diplopia

B. There is a noticeable hyphema in the affected eye

C. The patient reports photophobia and excessive tearing

D. The eye appears to protrude forward

120. Which of the following signs would suggest a possible basilar skull fracture in a patient with facial trauma?

    A. Clear fluid draining from the ear

    B. Subconjunctival hemorrhage

    C. Presence of a black eye

    D. Swelling over the zygomatic arch

121. When managing a patient with suspected neck injury due to blunt trauma, what is a priority?

    A. Providing pain relief medication

    B. Immobilization using a cervical collar and spine board

    C. Encouraging neck movements to assess range of motion

    D. Applying heat to reduce muscle spasms

122. What is the first step in managing chemical burns to both eyes?

    A. Cover both eyes with sterile dressings.

    B. Begin irrigation with clean water immediately.

    C. Administer an analgesic for pain management.

    D. Assess visual acuity prior to any intervention.

123. In cases of suspected spinal cord injury at the level of C5, what is an important aspect to monitor?

    A. Blood glucose levels

    B. Respiratory effectiveness

    C. Pupil reactivity

    D. Urinary output

124. When assessing a patient with maxillofacial trauma, what complication should be immediately addressed?

    A. Cosmetic disfigurement

    B. Airway obstruction

    C. Long-term mastication problems

    D. Difficulty swallowing

125. During the secondary assessment of a patient with blunt force trauma to the back, which symptom most strongly suggests spinal injury?

    A. Localized pain at the site of impact
    B. Loss of sensation in the extremities
    C. Bruising along the lumbar region
    D. Complaints of general back discomfort

126. What is the FIRST step in the assessment of a patient with suspected chest trauma?

    A. Check for a pulse
    B. Open the airway
    C. Perform a rapid scan for bleeding
    D. Apply oxygen

127. Which of the following is a sign of tension pneumothorax?

    A. Steady blood pressure
    B. Decreased breath sounds on one side
    C. Bilateral chest movement
    D. Pink, warm skin

128. What is the most appropriate management for an open chest wound?

    A. Tight bandage around the chest
    B. Application of cold packs to the injury site
    C. Immediate needle decompression
    D. Covering the wound with an occlusive dressing

129. Which of these symptoms most likely indicates severe abdominal trauma?

    A. Increased thirst
    B. Hyperactive bowel sounds
    C. Rigidity and guarding of the abdomen
    D. Coughing up a small amount of blood

130. How might shock present in a patient with a severe abdominal injury?

    A. Rapid, bounding pulse
    B. Slow respiratory rate
    C. Hypotension and tachycardia
    D. Hyperactive reflexes

131. Which diagnostic procedure is most commonly used at the scene to assess thoracic trauma?

    A. FAST ultrasound
    B. CT scan
    C. Chest X-ray
    D. Auscultation

132. In the case of a flail chest, what sign would you expect to find on physical examination?

    A. Paradoxical chest movement
    B. Unilateral chest pain
    C. Symmetrical chest expansion
    D. Clear and equal breath sounds

133. When assessing a pediatric patient who has suffered trauma, which of the following is an important consideration?

    A. A child's vital signs may appear normal even when in shock
    B. Pediatric patients are less likely to suffer multiple system injuries
    C. It is less important to maintain a pediatric patient's body temperature
    D. Head injuries are uncommon in pediatric trauma cases

134. In geriatric patients who have experienced trauma, why is it important to obtain a thorough medication history?

    A. They are less likely to be on any medications
    B. Medications can mask typical signs of injury and illness
    C. Most geriatric patients suffer from memory loss and need reminders on medication intake
    D. Medications have no impact on the treatment of trauma patients

135. When dealing with trauma in geriatric populations, what is the significance of recognizing "silent" heart attacks?

    A. Geriatric patients are less likely to experience heart attacks
    B. The atypical presentation of heart attacks in the elderly may complicate injury assessments
    C. Only young patients can have "silent" heart attacks
    D. Heart attacks in geriatric patients are always accompanied by chest pain

136. Which of the following interventions is typically NOT appropriate for a pediatric patient with suspected spinal injury?

   A. Immobilization using age-appropriate devices
   B. Log roll technique for positioning
   C. Application of a cervical collar that is appropriately sized for adults
   D. Backboarding if indicated by protocols or mechanism of injury

137. You arrive at a scene where an elderly patient has fallen. What key consideration should you keep in mind during your assessment?

   A. Elderly patients rarely sustain serious injuries from falls
   B. Elderly patients often have osteoporosis making fractures more likely
   C. It is uncommon for elderly patients to be taking anticoagulants
   D. Geriatric falls should be treated as low-priority incidents

138. When assessing a child after a motor vehicle collision, why is it important to pay particular attention to abdominal injuries?

   A. Abdominal injuries are easily identified in children
   B. Children's abdominal organs are better protected and rarely injured
   C. Abdominal wall muscles are less developed in children, making organ injury more likely without external signs
   D. The abdomen is usually not affected during vehicle collisions in pediatrics

139. When approaching a patient who has experienced multisystem trauma, what is the first step you should take?

   A. Obtain a detailed medical history
   B. Stabilize the cervical spine
   C. Begin transport to the nearest facility
   D. Administer pain medication

140. A patient has fallen from a significant height and is presenting with uneven chest rise, decreased breath sounds on the left side, and tracheal deviation. What is the most likely cause of these symptoms?

   A. Pneumonia
   B. Tension pneumothorax
   C. Hemothorax
   D. Rib fractures

141. You arrive at a car accident scene to find a driver with an open abdominal wound. Which of the following is an appropriate immediate action?

    A. Apply direct pressure to the wound.

    B. Attempt to replace any protruding organs.

    C. Provide oral fluids to prevent dehydration.

    D. Cover the wound with a sterile moist dressing and secure it with an occlusive dressing.

142. Upon assessing a patient with multisystem trauma, you note distended neck veins, muffled heart sounds, and hypotension. What condition should you suspect?

    A. Cardiac tamponade

    B. Myocardial contusion

    C. Pericarditis

    D. Congestive heart failure

143. A multisystem trauma patient with suspected pelvic fracture should be transported in which position?

    A. Supine with hips flexed and knees bent

    B. Prone to alleviate pressure on the pelvis

    C. Lateral recumbent (recovery position)

    D. Supine on a backboard with pelvic binder

144. You encounter a patient who was ejected from their vehicle during an accident. They are responsive but confused and have both upper extremity fractures and unstable vital signs. What is your best course of action?

    A. Immediate transport utilizing lights and sirens.

    B. Splint fractures on scene before transport for pain control.

    C. Take time to perform detailed secondary assessment before deciding on transport.

    D. Call for aeromedical evacuation due to severe nature of injuries.

145. What is the first step in the management of a patient with severe hypothermia who is found unconscious?

    A. Provide immediate CPR

    B. Apply passive external rewarming techniques

    C. Assess vitals and manage airway

    D. Start active internal rewarming

146. When treating a frostbite injury, which one of the following actions is generally advised against in pre-hospital care?

A. Gently rewarming the affected area

B. Massaging the frostbitten tissue

C. Protecting the tissue from further injury

D. Encouraging gentle movement of the affected extremity

147. What action should be taken first when managing a drowning victim who has been pulled from the water and is not breathing?

A. Transport immediately to hospital without interventions

B. Place the individual in recovery position to clear fluid from airway

C. Perform rescue breathing or CPR as necessary

D. Warm the victim by removing wet clothing and covering with blankets

148. For a conscious patient who has suffered from cold exposure with no immediate danger present, what is an appropriate care technique?

A. Encourage intake of hot caffeinated beverages to aid in warming

B. Initiate rapid active internal rewarming

C. Offer warm sweetened liquids, if able to swallow safely

D. Keep patient stationary and wait for emergency medical services without intervention

149. A lightning strike victim is unconscious but breathing with a weak pulse. Which one is NOT a priority in this scenario?

A. Maintaining cervical spine stabilization

B. Monitoring for cardiac arrhythmias

C. Administering oxygen therapy

D. Checking for exit wounds before assessing airway and breathing

150. What immediate danger exists for someone exposed to extremely cold water temperatures, besides hypothermia?

A. Heat stroke due to quick temperature changes when rescued

B. Cold water shock potentially leading to cardiac arrest

C. Dehydration because they might not feel the need to drink water

D. Frostbite since cold water increases its likelihood rapidly

Answer Key with Detailed Explanations

1. D: Typically, during a myocardial infarction, the patient may experience hypotension due to the heart's reduced capability to pump blood efficiently, not hypertension.

2. C: Patients with CHF may experience acute pulmonary edema, so high flow oxygen therapy is essential to improve hypoxia. Nitroglycerin may also be used but after oxygen is initiated.

3. B: The ECG findings suggest ventricular fibrillation (VF), which is a shockable rhythm. The immediate course of action should be defibrillation.

4. B: Nitroglycerin can cause hypotension; therefore, it should be administered with caution in patients who have low blood pressure or are on medications for erectile dysfunction.

5. C: In a hypertensive emergency, the primary goal is to prevent organ damage by reducing blood pressure gradually; lowering it too quickly can result in ischemia.

6. B: Torsades de Pointes is characterized by its distinctive pattern on an ECG where the QRS complexes appear to twist around the isoelectric line.

7. C: Aspirin helps prevent platelet aggregation and reduces mortality in AMI patients.

8. B: VF is a life-threatening arrhythmia that requires immediate defibrillation.

9. A: In a tension pneumothorax, accumulation of air in the pleural space can cause shift of the mediastinum and tracheal deviation away from the affected side. This is a grave sign and requires immediate intervention.

10. A: A patient experiencing asthma will often have prolonged expiratory phase and wheezing due to bronchoconstriction. Stridor is usually associated with upper airway obstructions, not asthma.

11. B: CPAP (continuous positive airway pressure) is often used for patients with congestive heart failure (CHF), evidenced by frothy sputum as it forces fluid back into the pulmonary circulation.

12. B: Oxygen administration and prompt transport to a hospital are critical in suspected pulmonary embolism so that definitive care and diagnostics can be provided.

13. A: Flail chest results in paradoxical movement — the flail segment moves inwards on inspiration and outwards on expiration — because it's not stabilized by intact ribs.

14. A: These signs are indicative of asthma exacerbation, which can lead to reduced air exchange and increased work of breathing, necessitating a tripod position to aid respiration.

15. B: These are classic signs of cardiac tamponade, known as Beck's triad; they indicate fluid accumulation in the pericardium impeding cardiac output.

16. C: Hyperventilation syndrome typically does not cause pinpoint pupils. It is more often associated with symptoms such as carpopedal spasm, tachycardia, and numbness or tingling in the extremities due to respiratory alkalosis.

17. C: Slurred speech is a common sign of a stroke, as it can result from the disruption of normal nerve function in the brain affecting speech control.

18. C: The combination of severe headache, photophobia, and neck stiffness is highly suggestive of subarachnoid hemorrhage rather than other types of headaches.

19. B: Assessing the level of consciousness using the Glasgow Coma Scale is critical for determining the severity of a traumatic brain injury.

20. C: Ensuring an open airway and positioning them safely are first-line responses to manage generalized tonic-clonic seizures.

21. A: Early administration of antibiotics can be life-saving in cases of bacterial meningitis.

22. C: An epidural hematoma often presents with hemiparesis due to its impact on one hemisphere that controls motor function on one side of the body.

23. B: While confusion and aggression can have many causes, in the context of trauma from a motor vehicle collision, intracerebral hemorrhage must be considered.

24. B: Sudden onset paralysis on one side is indicative of ischemic stroke, particularly in older individuals with risk factors such as hypertension.

25. C: A patient experiencing an abdominal aortic aneurysm often presents with a tearing sensation and may exhibit a pulsating mass in the abdomen. This is due to the enlargement and potential rupture of the abdominal aorta.

26. A: The sudden onset of sharp, epigastric pain radiating to the back, particularly in a patient with heavy alcohol use, is very indicative of acute pancreatitis.

27. C: Classic symptoms of appendicitis include sudden-onset right lower quadrant (RLQ) pain, fever, and rebound tenderness.

28. C: Melena is characterized by black, tarry stools which typically indicates bleeding higher up in the gastrointestinal tract, such as from the stomach or small intestine.

29. B: Severe epigastric pain associated with signs of shock such as pale skin, anxiety, tachycardia, and hypotension suggests a possible perforated peptic ulcer.

30. C: Symptoms that are alleviated by eating food or antacids but recur later are characteristic of peptic ulcer disease.

31. C: Acute cholecystitis typically presents with sudden, intense pain in the upper right abdominal quadrant, which can radiate to the back or right shoulder, often triggered by fatty meal consumption.

32. B: With prolonged vomiting and diarrhea leading to severe dehydration, loss of potassium is common, putting the patient at risk of hypokalemia.

33. C: Type 1 diabetes mellitus is characterized by the absence or minimal production of insulin by the pancreas, necessitating insulin therapy.

34. B: Polydipsia, or excessive thirst, is a typical early sign of HHS that results from the body's attempt to counteract high blood glucose by increasing fluid intake.

35. C: For an unresponsive diabetic patient, it is vital to first check their blood glucose level to determine if they are hypoglycemic or hyperglycemic before initiating appropriate treatment.

36. D: Infection or intense stress can raise hormonal levels that counteract insulin, leading to high blood sugar and development of DKA.

37. C: During treatment for DKA, potassium levels often drop rapidly and can lead to life-threatening hypokalemia which needs to be corrected carefully.

38. C: Thyroid storm is associated with symptoms like fever and tachycardia due to an excess of thyroid hormones; these symptoms contrast starkly with the slow metabolic features of hypothyroidism.

39. C: A conscious patient who can swallow safely should be given oral glucose preparations as it's a fast-acting source of sugar for reversing hypoglycemia.

40. A: Untreated hypoglycemia can lead to loss of consciousness, seizures, and if prolonged without treatment, potentially to diabetic coma.

41. D: Hives (urticaria) and itching (pruritus) are common signs of an allergic reaction and can indicate a systemic reaction.

42. C: Intramuscular epinephrine is the first-line treatment for anaphylaxis due to its rapid onset of action in counteracting the symptoms.

43. B: Difficulty breathing and swelling around the neck after an insect sting are signs of an anaphylactic reaction.

44. B: Patients with known allergies exposed to their specific allergen are at greatest risk for developing anaphylaxis.

45. B: Patients often express feelings of dread or a sense that something is seriously wrong, which can precede more definitive signs of allergic reactions and anaphylaxis.

46. B: Oxygen therapy can help manage respiratory distress resulting from allergic reactions or anaphylaxis.

47. D: The correct "Five Rights" include the right patient, right medication, right dose, right route, and right time; ensuring medication has not expired is important but it's not classically listed as one of the Five Rights.

48. B: Securing the airway is crucial in anaphylaxis management due to the risk of airway compromise from swelling and bronchoconstriction.

49. B: Withdrawal from alcohol can result in severe depressive symptoms, unlike stimulants like cocaine and methamphetamine which typically cause rebound depression shortly after the effects wear off, or opioids like heroin which lead to physical withdrawal symptoms.

50. D: The antidote for acetaminophen (Tylenol) overdose is acetylcysteine, which helps to replenish glutathione reserves and protect the liver from damage.

51. B: Opioid overdose commonly results in pinpoint pupils (miosis), along with respiratory depression and decreased levels of consciousness.

52. B: Amphetamine is a stimulant that increases activity in the central nervous system, leading to increased wakefulness and activity, among other effects.

53. B: Benzodiazepines are central nervous system depressants and can lead to significant respiratory depression in overdose situations.

54. B: Tolerance occurs when someone needs larger doses of a drug to achieve the same level of intoxication or effect that they previously achieved with smaller amounts due to repeated use.

55. C: Activated charcoal is not indicated when corrosive substances are ingested because it does not adsorb these materials and can worsen their caustic effects on the gastrointestinal tract.

56. A: Flumazenil is a benzodiazepine antagonist and can be used to treat benzodiazepine overdoses by reversing their sedative effects.

57. A: Because heat stroke is best treated by rapidly cooling the body, and applying cool packs to areas with large blood vessels aids in reducing core temperature.

58. B: Because anaphylaxis often causes bronchoconstriction, leading to wheezing on both inspiration and expiration.

59. C: Rapid rewarming can cause further tissue damage; instead gently warming and protecting from further cold exposure is recommended.

60. A: Applying ice can cause local vasoconstriction which may concentrate venom in one area increasing tissue damage.

61. B: Dry clothing and blankets will help reduce further heat loss without causing any potential harm that could occur from other suggested methods.

62. A: Carbon monoxide binds with hemoglobin more effectively than oxygen does; administering high-flow oxygen helps displace carbon monoxide from hemoglobin molecules.

63. B: Decompression sickness occurs when nitrogen bubbles form in the blood and tissues when a diver ascends too quickly. Treatment includes breathing 100% oxygen and undergoing hyperbaric recompression therapy to reduce bubbles.

64. C: Minimizing contact with the ground and staying low while avoiding tall structures or conductive materials reduces the risk of being struck by lightning.

65. C: Tuberculosis is an infectious disease caused by the bacterium Mycobacterium tuberculosis. It primarily affects the lungs and is transmitted through airborne particles from an infected person when they cough or sneeze.

66. C: Decreased urine output can be an indication of severe sepsis, which may lead to poor organ perfusion and eventually multiple organ dysfunction syndrome (MODS).

67. A: Hepatitis A virus is often spread through ingesting contaminated food or water. It's less likely to cause chronic liver disease compared to some other forms of hepatitis.

68. D: Meningococcal meningitis is highly contagious and can be transmitted through respiratory droplets. Full barrier precautions including gloves, gown, face shield, and N95 mask should be used to protect against infection.

69. B: Fever, headache, and particularly a stiff neck are classic signs of meningitis—an inflammation of the protective membranes covering the brain and spinal cord.

70. D: HIV is commonly transmitted through certain bodily fluids including blood, semen, vaginal fluids, rectal fluids, and breast milk—but not through sweat or tears.

71. C: After exposure to the influenza virus, individuals generally show symptoms after 1 to 4 days during the incubation period as the virus replicates.

72. C: The Ebola virus disease has a high mortality rate; early recognition can improve survival chances due to supportive care being initiated quickly. Additionally, early identification allows for proper isolation measures to prevent community spread. Antibiotics are not effective since Ebola is viral.

73. B: Establishing a therapeutic rapport and ensuring the scene is safe are primary concerns when approaching a patient with a psychiatric emergency. This sets the foundation for effective communication and assessment, while also addressing safety for all parties involved.

74. D: Maintaining a calm demeanor and using active listening skills can help de-escalate a potentially volatile situation by showing empathy and respect towards the patient's feelings and emotions.

75. B: Haloperidol is an antipsychotic medication that is often utilized as chemical restraint to help control severely agitated patients during psychiatric emergencies.

76. C: When necessary, restraints should be used to ensure safety; however, they must be applied correctly to avoid compromising circulation and respiration.

77. B: Inquiring about the presence of an elaborate plan can help evaluate suicide risk by determining if there is an immediate threat requiring urgent intervention.

78. C: Substance abuse can cause panic attacks due to alterations made by substances within brain chemistry, which may result in increased anxiety levels and panic symptoms.

79. D: Bystanders should give emergency personnel space to work and follow instructions so that professionals can manage the situation without additional stress or interference.

80. C: EMS providers are required by law to maintain confidentiality and protect patients' personal health information in adherence with HIPAA regulations.

81. C: Preeclampsia is a pregnancy complication characterized by high blood pressure and signs of damage to another organ system, often the kidneys, which is indicated by proteinuria. Edema (swelling) is also common. However, hyperreflexia rather than hyporeflexia is typically associated with preeclampsia.

82. D: The first-line management for postpartum hemorrhage includes uterine massage to stimulate contractions and help stop bleeding. Checking for retained placental parts is crucial as their presence can prevent uterine contraction and exacerbate bleeding.

83. B: Vaginal bleeding combined with a positive pregnancy test can be indicative of an ectopic pregnancy, especially when accompanied by signs such as unilateral pelvic pain. Ectopic pregnancy occurs when a fertilized egg implants outside the uterus, often in one of the fallopian tubes, which can cause life-threatening bleeding if not identified and treated promptly.

84. C: In cases of umbilical cord prolapse, it is important to relieve pressure on the cord to maintain oxygen supply to the fetus. Positioning the mother so that her hips are elevated or she is in knee-chest position can reduce pressure on the cord until medical intervention can take place.

85. C: Managing gestational diabetes involves careful monitoring of maternal blood glucose levels and maintaining a balanced diet tailored for diabetes management. Regular consultations with healthcare providers are also crucial to adjust treatment as needed and to assess for complications.

86. B: Ovarian torsion is an emergency condition that requires prompt surgical intervention to preserve ovarian function. Delayed treatment can lead to ischemia and necrosis of the ovary due to disrupted blood supply.

87. A: Placenta previa is characterized by sudden, painless vaginal bleeding in the second or third trimester due to the placenta covering the cervical opening. It is diagnosed through ultrasound rather than clinical symptoms alone, as it can mimic other conditions.

88. C: The initial step in managing shoulder dystocia, where one of the baby's shoulders becomes stuck behind the mother's pelvic bone during delivery, is applying suprapubic pressure. This helps rotate the fetus's shoulder into a more favorable position and facilitates delivery while minimizing risk to both mother and infant. Fundal pressure is contraindicated as it can worsen the impaction.

89. C: Direct pressure with a clean cloth or dressing is the initial step in controlling bleeding before considering other interventions such as elevation or tourniquet application.

90. B: Covering the wound with a flutter-valve dressing (occlusive dressing that allows air to escape but not enter) helps prevent air from entering the pleural space while letting existing air escape.

91. B: Cold and clammy skin can be indicative of internal bleeding and may signify shock due to blood loss even without visible bleeding.

92. C: Ecchymosis refers to the blue or purplish discoloration of the skin caused by the leakage of blood into surrounding tissue.

93. D: Wrapped in dry sterile gauze and placed in a plastic bag kept cool with ice provides an optimal environment for preserving an amputated part during transport without causing further tissue damage from direct contact with ice.

94. C: A tourniquet is indicated for an extremity injury where life-threatening bleeding cannot be controlled by direct pressure or dressings.

95. A: Compartment syndrome is a critical condition that can occur following severe soft tissue trauma, characterized by increased pressure within a closed muscle compartment, compromising blood flow and tissue viability.

96. B: Flushing the affected area with large amounts of water dilutes and washes away the chemical, which is essential in the initial management of chemical burns to minimize tissue damage.

97. B: Airway patency is always the first priority in trauma patients, including those with burns, to ensure they can breathe.

98. C: Elevation helps reduce swelling, and covering burns with a dry, sterile dressing helps prevent infection.

99. A: The severity of burns is influenced by factors like age, preexisting conditions, size (percentage of Total Body Surface Area - TBSA), depth, and location of burns.

100. D: The Rule of Nines and Lund and Browder chart are both appropriate methods for estimating TBSA in burn patients.

101. C: Full-thickness burns penetrate all layers of skin and often require surgical intervention like skin grafting for treatment.

102. C: Removing contaminated clothing is crucial to stop further chemical exposure before flushing the skin with water.

103. C: Sooty sputum or singed nasal hairs indicate an inhalation injury which commonly accompanies facial or neck burns.

104. C: Electrical burns often cause more internal damage than can be seen on the surface due to electricity traveling through tissues.

105. A: Before immobilization, it is critical to assess for distal pulses, motor function, and sensory function in the injured extremity; however, the most immediate action for a femur fracture is immobilization with a traction splint to stabilize the fracture and prevent further injury.

106. C: While both dislocations and fractures can present with pain, bruising, and potentially lost pulses if severe enough, visible deformity at the joint typically suggests a dislocation where the bone ends are no longer in their normal positions.

107. B: For musculoskeletal injuries such as suspect wrist fractures from falls, it's best to splint them in the position you find them. Attempting to move or realign injuries could cause further damage. Checking for a pulse is important but comes after immobilizing as not to exacerbate any damage during assessment.

108. C: Always check neurovascular status (distal pulses, sensation, and movement below injury), which will impact further treatment decisions. Do not attempt to realign; this is handled by hospital personnel unless there are specific life-threatening circumstances which mandate field intervention.

109. C: A sprain refers specifically to an injury involving ligaments (which connect bone to bone), typically occurring from overstretching or tearing due to unnatural movements or forces applied to a joint -- unlike strains which refer to muscle or tendon injuries.

110. C: The R.I.C.E method is a widely accepted initial treatment for soft tissue injuries such as sprains. It helps in minimizing swelling and discomfort. Heat should not be applied initially as it can worsen swelling, and walking on a sprained ankle could cause further injury.

111. C: While physical symptoms such as tenderness, deformity, and neurovascular impairment are indicative of fractures, an X-ray is essential for confirming a fracture diagnosis as it provides clear imaging of bone integrity and alignment.

112. D: An irregular breathing pattern, such as Cheyne-Stokes respiration or ataxic (Biot's) respirations, can be an indicator of increased intracranial pressure affecting the brain stem.

113. B: The jaw-thrust maneuver without head extension is used to open the airway in patients with suspected spinal injury to avoid further spinal cord damage.

114. A: Clear fluid draining from the nose or ears (cerebrospinal fluid rhinorrhea or otorrhea) could suggest a basilar skull fracture, which is a serious head injury.

115. B: Immediate manual immobilization of the spine is critical in this scenario to prevent potential secondary injury due to movement.

116. C: Bruising around the eyes (raccoon eyes) and behind the ears (Battle's sign) are indicative of a basilar skull fracture, which is a severe injury at the base of the skull.

117. A: Priapism, which is an involuntary erection in males, can be an indicator of spinal cord injury, typically reflecting damage at or below T7.

118. B: To assess motor function without aggravating a suspected cervical spine injury, asking patients to move their hands and fingers avoids moving their neck or back but still provides information on motor function integrity.

119. B: While all of these symptoms can be concerning, a hyphema, or pooling of blood in the anterior chamber of the eye, can indicate serious injury to internal eye structures and lead to permanent vision impairment. It is considered an emergency that requires immediate medical intervention.

120. A: Clear fluid draining from the ear or nose can be indicative of cerebrospinal fluid leak associated with a basilar skull fracture which is often a result of high-impact injuries to the head and may accompany serious brain injuries.

121. B: Immobilization is crucial in suspected neck injuries to prevent further damage to the cervical spine, which could lead to paralysis or other neurological deficits.

122. B: Immediate irrigation is essential for chemical burns to dilute and remove the caustic substance and reduce tissue damage; delaying this intervention can result in more severe injury or blindness.

123. B: A spinal cord injury at or above C5 can impair diaphragm function due to possible paralysis of respiratory muscles; monitoring respiratory effectiveness is critical as it could quickly become life-threatening.

124. B: Airway obstruction is an immediate life-threat. Maxillofacial trauma can cause bleeding, swelling, or tissue displacement that may obstruct the airway and requires prompt attention.

125. B: Loss of sensation or paralysis in the extremities may indicate damage to the spinal cord or nerve roots, emblematic of a spinal injury. This necessitates prompt and careful immobilization and transport.

126. B: The initial assessment of any trauma patient begins with ensuring an adequate airway, as per the ABC (Airway, Breathing, Circulation) priority sequence in trauma care.

127. B: Decreased or absent breath sounds on one side of the chest is a classic sign of tension pneumothorax due to lung collapse on the affected side.

128. D: An occlusive dressing prevents air from being sucked into the chest cavity during inhalation, reducing the risk of developing a tension pneumothorax.

129. C: Rigidity and guarding are signs of irritation or inflammation in the abdominal cavity, often associated with serious injuries.

130. C: Hypotension (low blood pressure) and tachycardia (rapid heart rate) are common signs of hemorrhagic shock, which can occur with severe abdominal injuries leading to internal bleeding.

131. D: While CT scans and X-rays are more definitive, auscultation—listening to chest sounds—is commonly used at the scene for immediate assessment.

132. A: Paradoxical movement—where part of the chest moves in with inhalation and out with exhalation—is indicative of a flail chest, where multiple adjacent ribs are fractured in more than one place.

133. A: Children can compensate for shock longer than adults and may maintain normal vital signs until their condition suddenly deteriorates.

134. B: The elderly often take multiple medications that can alter their physiological response to trauma, masking typical signs.

135. B: Elderly patients often have atypical symptoms during a myocardial infarction, which can complicate the assessment and may be confused with other traumatic injuries.

136. C: An adult-sized cervical collar will not properly immobilize a pediatric patient's spine due to the different proportions of their anatomy.

137. B: Due to conditions like osteoporosis, elderly people are more prone to fractures from falls than younger individuals.

138. C: Children have less developed protective muscle mass so significant internal injury can occur with minimal or no external injury indicators.

139. B: In any trauma situation, especially multisystem trauma, the priority is to stabilize the cervical spine to prevent any potential spinal cord injury.

140. B: Uneven chest rise, decreased breath sounds on one side, and tracheal deviation are classic signs of tension pneumothorax, a life-threatening condition often caused by trauma.

141. D: For open abdominal wounds, cover with a sterile moist dressing and then an occlusive dressing to prevent contamination and further injury; do not apply pressure or push back any protruding organs.

142. A: Beck's triad (distended neck veins, muffled heart sounds, hypotension) indicates cardiac tamponade; this condition can occur following chest trauma and requires immediate intervention.

143. D: Patients with suspected pelvic fractures should be immobilized in a supine position on a backboard; if available, a pelvic binder can help limit internal bleeding and movement of fracture segments.

144. A: The patient is displaying signs of possible traumatic brain injury as well as shock; they require rapid transport for advanced care while performing en route splinting as necessary.

145. C: The primary concern should always be to manage the airway and circulatory status of an unconscious patient while protecting their spine, particularly for those suspected of severe hypothermia.

146. B: Massaging frostbitten tissues can cause further damage to already compromised tissues and is not recommended.

147. C: Immediate assessment of breathing and circulation, followed by rescue breathing or CPR if needed, are critical for survival in drowning victims.

148. C: Providing warm sweetened liquids can help increase internal body temperature if there's no risk of aspiration.

149. D: While exit wounds are significant findings in lightning injuries, assessing and managing airway and breathing are immediate priorities over wound examination.

150. B: Cold water shock can cause an involuntary gasp response upon sudden immersion, followed by hyperventilation, which can ultimately lead to cardiac arrest even before significant hypothermia develops.

Unlock Your NREMT Exam Success with an Exclusive Free Bonus!

Dear Aspiring EMT,

Thank you for choosing our NREMT Exam Preparation Guide! We are thrilled to support your journey to becoming a Nationally Registered Emergency Medical Technician.

Unlock Your Path to Success with a Single Scan!

Gear up to excel in your NREMT exam with our exclusive bonus: "NREMT Exam Prep: 650 Questions and Answers" eBook. This comprehensive resource is crafted to enhance your understanding and elevate your confidence as you approach your examination day. And the best part? Instant access is just a QR code scan away!

Go Green, Go Digital!

By opting for our digital bonus, you're not only preparing for your exam efficiently but also contributing to environmental conservation. This eco-friendly option helps minimize paper use, reducing pollution and saving trees. Together, we're not just striving for academic success; we're also fostering a healthier planet.

Key Benefits:
- Access to over 650 meticulously designed questions and answers.
- Instant availability on your device, enabling you to study anytime, anywhere.
- A sustainable, eco-friendly approach to your exam preparation.

Here's How to Claim Your Bonus:
1. Open the camera on your phone.
2. Point it at the QR code below.
3. Tap the notification to download your "NREMT Exam Prep: 650 Questions and Answers" eBook.

It's that easy! Get ready to excel in your NREMT exam and make a positive impact on the environment. Your path to a successful career in emergency medical services is just a scan away!

CHAPTER 12

MASTERING NREMT SKILLS STATIONS

Preparing for Practical Examinations

Entering into a NREMT practical examination without the right preparation is like walking into a minefield blindfolded. It's imperative that candidates approach these exams with a clear strategy and thorough preparation. When it comes to preparing, consider starting with a self-assessment. Review each skill in your study guide, and honestly rate your proficiency. Identify the areas where you feel least confident, and prioritize them in your study schedule.

Next up is practice—and we're not talking about a casual walk-through of procedures. This needs to be deliberate practice, which involves setting specific goals, receiving immediate feedback, and concentrating on technique until actions become second nature. Join study groups or partner with peers to simulate exam conditions as closely as possible. Engage in role-playing scenarios to heighten your comfort level with the unpredictability of patient responses.

Maintain an inventory checklist for each skill station to ensure you walk in prepared with every required item memorized or readily on hand where allowed. Moreover, never underestimate the power of studying the NREMT skill sheets provided for each station. They outline critical fail points and exact steps evaluators expect to see demonstrated competently.

Mental preparation carries just as much weight as physical preparation. Visualizing success can enhance confidence levels dramatically. Practice mindfulness techniques to manage stress and retain focus during the actual exam.

Step-by-Step Skill Station Guides

When tackling individual skills stations, having a bulletproof approach helps prevent errors under pressure. Imagine each station as a scene where you're both the director and lead actor; control what you can to render an impeccable performance.

For instance, in Airway/Respiration/Ventilation skills station, the basis of every intervention is ensuring patent airways and effective ventilation. You must be able to select appropriate airway adjuncts such as oral or nasal airways and utilize suction techniques competently.

If faced with a Cardiac Arrest Management/AED station, timing is key; precision in delivering compressions, breaths, and timely defibrillation could be what stands between life or death. Familiarity with AED operation is crucial here—practice until the sequence becomes instinctive.

In Patient Assessment stations, you'll demonstrate your ability to conduct systematic assessments (medical/trauma) with an emphasis on scene safety, initial assessment, physical examinations, patient history collection (SAMPLE), and proper communication (both patient reporting and documentation). While performing Spinal Immobilization or Long Bone Fracture stations require meticulous attention to immobilization techniques without causing further harm to the patient.

For Obstetrics/Gynecological stations involving childbirth scenarios, readiness means more than just knowing stages of labor—it's about ensuring mother's and baby's safety through proper delivery technique management of complications such as breech presentation or cord prolapse. Similarly, treating bleeding control and shock management requires you not only stop the bleeding through direct pressure but also recognize signs of shock early and initiate appropriate interventions.

Remember that psychomotor skills are just one aspect of patient care; they must be combined with strong communication skills for effective verbal reports during each station exam. Always re-assess your work before concluding any given station; have you followed all necessary steps without taking shortcuts? Have you ensured patient comfort throughout the procedure? Never leave any room for doubt that you have provided optimum patient care according to NREMT standards.

Common Mistakes and How to Avoid Them

The pathway to mastery involves learning from mistakes—both yours and others'. Be aware of the common pitfalls encountered by candidates at different NREMT skills stations so that you may sidestep them.

1. **Skipping Steps:** Under stress, candidates often forget critical steps in a sequence. To avoid this, deepen your familiarity with each skill so that every step becomes second nature.

2. **Poor Communication:** Communication issues can disrupt patient assessment or obscuration of important findings—always remember to clearly verbalize what you are doing and what you are observing.

3. **Overlooking Scene Safety:** Never begin patient care without first ensuring scene safety, even during simulations; evaluators are keen on this aspect.

4. **Misusing Equipment:** Incorrect application or operation of EMS tools can lead to automatic failure; revisit how each piece should be properly used during your study sessions.

5. **Lack of Confidence:** Demonstrate decisiveness in your actions; hesitation could suggest uncertainty about proper procedures which might affect an evaluator's perception of your competence.

6. **Ignoring Standard Precautions:** Always follow standard precautions without being prompted—such as applying gloves when necessary—to emphasize patient safety and your understanding of contamination risks.

7. **Inadequate Patient Assessment & Documentation:** Make sure to perform full patient assessments and notate key findings; skipping details could result in missed critical information impacting patient care scenarios.

CHAPTER 13

TEST-TAKING STRATEGIES FOR SUCCESS

Understanding the Exam Format

Embracing the format of your NREMT exam is the foremost step towards test-taking success. The National Registry of Emergency Medical Technicians (NREMT) examination is a computer-based, adaptive test that meticulously evaluates your understanding and abilities. The key to mastering this exam starts with recognizing the type of questions and the structure you will encounter.

The NREMT exam presents a series of multiple-choice questions designed with one best answer. It's crucial to realize that this adaptive test adjusts its difficulty based on your responses. Answering a question correctly will typically lead to a slightly more challenging question, whereas an incorrect answer will bring up an easier question. The goal of the exam is to determine your level of competence across five major areas: Airway, Respiration & Ventilation; Cardiology & Resuscitation; Trauma; Medical & Obstetrics/Gynecology; and EMS Operations.

As you study, familiarize yourself with the outline provided by the NREMT which details the topics and subtopics you'll need to master. Understanding this blueprint is much more effective than trying to memorize textbook content verbatim. Also, consider the standard length and timing of the test. While it varies for each candidate, prepare mentally for an exam that might have as many as 70 to 120 questions and can last up to two hours.

Strategies for Answering Multiple-Choice Questions

Succeeding in multiple-choice scenarios necessitates strategic thinking alongside your emergency medical knowledge. Here are some strategies to optimize your chances:

1. Read every question carefully. The nuances in wording can sometimes be subtle but critical in discerning what is actually being asked. Avoid skimming through the questions or answers too hastily, as important details might be missed.

2. Always aim to identify keywords or phrases within a question—these can provide hints about the most accurate answer or help eliminate incorrect options. Similarly, watch out for qualifiers such as "always," "never," "only," or "most." These words can drastically change a statement's meaning and often signal that an option may be entirely too absolute to be the best answer.

3. When faced with exceptionally challenging questions, apply what you've learned about patient care priorities. Think about scene safety, primary assessments, and immediate life-threatening conditions when determining what action should be taken first in any given scenario. This approach aligns with NREMT's philosophy and allows you to prioritize effectively under pressure.

4. Do not rush through the exam; instead, manage your time prudently. Spend a reasonable amount on each question but do not linger excessively if you are unsure about an answer. Mark it for review if this feature is available and move on—sometimes later questions can jog your memory or provide context that helps with earlier ones.

5. Make educated guesses rather than choosing at random when you don't know an answer outright. By excluding one or two options that are clearly incorrect, you can significantly increase your odds of selecting the right one.

6. It's also crucial not to second-guess yourself incessantly—frequent changes from initial answers often result in switching from right choices to wrong ones. Trust in your training and intuition unless new information specifically justifies changing an answer.

Ensure you are fundamentally sound on common distractors used in multiple-choice exams such as similar sounding medications or conditions that have distinct differences. Detail-oriented studying will make these distinctions clearer during the actual exam.

Dealing with Exam Anxiety and Stress

At some point, nearly every test-taker feels some degree of anxiety or stress—and when it comes to high-stakes exams like the NREMT, those feelings can intensify. However, allowing stress and anxiety to take control can hinder your ability to concentrate and diminish your confidence.

The first step in managing test anxiety is preparation. When you're familiar with the content and comfortable with the format of the exam, much of the anxiety naturally dissipates. Create a study plan that covers all areas of knowledge required by the NREMT, and stick to it with discipline.

Another effective strategy is simulating examination conditions while practicing. Time yourself as you go through practice tests so you can become accustomed to the pressure of answering within certain time constraints.

Practicing relaxation techniques such as deep breathing exercises or mindfulness meditation can significantly reduce stress levels and improve focus when practiced regularly leading up to your exam date. A typical technique involves taking slow breaths while counting to five during both inhalation and exhalation, enabling your heart rate and mind to settle.

On test day, nourish your body and mind: eat a well-balanced breakfast for sustained energy levels without heavy foods that could make you drowsy. Dress comfortably in layers so you can adjust according to the temperature in the testing center. Arrive early so that you're not feeling rushed; being calm before starting your exam is essential for maintaining control over your nerves.

Maintain positive thoughts about your capabilities; self-confidence can actually lead to improved performance on an exam due to reduced anxiety levels. Remembering this might help: *"You have prepared for this; you understand how tests work; now it's just about showing what you know."*

CHAPTER 14

AFTER THE EXAM: NEXT STEPS

Interpreting Your NREMT Results

You've finally completed your National Registry of Emergency Medical Technicians (NREMT) exam—an admirable milestone in your journey towards a career in emergency medical services (EMS). However, the journey doesn't end here. After the exam, it's crucial to understand what your results mean and the next steps to take, regardless of whether you've passed or have to retake the test.

The NREMT provides a detailed score report for all test-takers, which gives you insight into your performance. Passing the NREMT is typically binary—you either pass or fail. If you receive a passing score, congratulations are in order! You are now eligible to be nationally certified as an EMT, which is a significant stepping stone for your career.

For those who do not pass on the first attempt, don't be discouraged. The NREMT provides candidates with a breakdown of their scores in various categories. This allows you to see areas where you performed well, alongside those where you may need further study and practice.

Understanding the results is simple: The score report will highlight your strengths and weaknesses across different content areas such as airway, respiration & ventilation;

cardiology & resuscitation; trauma; medical/obstetrics/gynecology, and more. If you see "above passing," it means you answered these questions correctly at a level beyond the minimum standard. "Near passing" indicates that you were close to the threshold, while "below passing" signifies that you need considerable improvement in that area.

Beginning your analysis here allows you to understand where your knowledge base stands and which areas will require more focus if a retake is necessary.

Remediation Strategies for a Retake

If you need to retake the NREMT exam, don't view it as a setback but as an opportunity to solidify and expand your knowledge base. You'll be more prepared than ever before on your second attempt with proper remediation.

Creating a study plan based on your results is essential. Focus on areas marked *"below passing,"* dedicating more time and resources to those subjects. Utilizing different study materials can also help reinforce learning—try interactive study aids like apps or flashcards if traditional textbooks weren't sufficient previously.

Joining study groups or finding study partners can provide multiple perspectives on challenging topics and keep motivation high. Additionally, consider reaching out to instructors or knowledgeable peers who can offer clarification on complex concepts you're struggling with.

Some tangible steps include:

1. **Revisiting Course Materials:** Go back through your EMT course syllabus and reread chapters related to your weak areas.
2. **Practice Tests:** Take numerous practice tests mimicking the NREMT's computer adaptive test environment.
3. **Skill Refreshers:** Reinforce practical skills by revisiting skills labs or using online simulations.
4. **Educational Videos/Podcasts:** Supplement reading materials with educational videos or podcasts that focus on emergency medical care.
5. **Professional Tutoring:** If possible, seek tutoring from experienced EMS educators.
6. **Rest and Self-Care:** While studying hard is vital, rest is equally important for cognitive retention and overall well-being.

When ready for a retake, approach the exam with confidence—remembering that this time around, you have an even greater understanding of what's expected due to your prior experience.

Transitioning from EMT Student to EMT Professional

Passing the NREMT and gaining certification is a pivotal moment in any EMT's career; however, remember that it is merely the beginning. As a certified EMT, it's now time to move forward and embrace the responsibilities of your new career with enthusiasm and professionalism.

Transitioning from student to workplace professional means more than just changing titles; it involves building upon all that you've learned and applying those skills in real-world scenarios. You'll make decisions that impact people's lives, so continuous learning and skill refinement are crucial. *Here are essential steps to ensure a smooth transition:*

1. **Secure Employment:** Begin applying for positions before graduation if possible but intensify your search once certified. Keep in mind that some regions have higher demands for EMTs than others.

2. **Ongoing Education:** Stay ahead by pursuing additional certifications such as Advanced Cardiac Life Support (ACLS) or Pediatric Advanced Life Support (PALS). These can improve job prospects and provide better care for patients.

3. **Skill Practice:** Regularly review practical skills and stay informed about new procedures or equipment within the field of emergency medicine.

4. **Join Professional Organizations:** Associations like The National Association of Emergency Medical Technicians (NAEMT) offer resources for continued education, networking opportunities, and staying updated on industry standards.

5. **Mental Resilience:** Working as an EMT can be emotionally taxing. Develop coping strategies such as peer support programs or professional counseling services to stay mentally fit for duty.

6. **Peer Connections:** Establish relationships with seasoned professionals who can provide mentorship and share their insights and experiences in EMS work.

7. **Personal Health:** Keep yourself physically fit – being an EMT is demanding – stamina is an asset when performing lifesaving procedures or lifting patients.

As exciting as it is daunting, transitioning into a professional role invites not only immense personal growth but also offers a chance to contribute significantly to society by ensuring public safety and health care delivery at its frontlines.

CHAPTER 15
CONTINUING EDUCATION AND PROFESSIONAL GROWTH

Lifelong Learning as an EMT

Emergency Medical Technicians (EMTs) are invaluable components of the healthcare field, responding to crises and providing critical care in people's most dire moments. However, after initial certification, the learning journey for an EMT is far from over. Lifelong learning is crucial for keeping skills sharp, staying current with medical advancements, and ensuring the best possible care for patients.

Continuing education in the EMT field often involves a myriad of approaches, including attending workshops, taking additional coursework, renewing certifications, and participating in hands-on skills training. These educational activities ensure that EMTs remain competent in life-saving techniques and patient assessment procedures. Moreover, they provide information on new equipment or methods that may emerge as technology and medical knowledge evolve.

Another essential aspect of lifelong learning for EMTs is remaining informed about the changing policies and protocols from local and national governing bodies like the National

Registry of Emergency Medical Technicians (NREMT). Updating oneself about these policies can be accomplished through official communications or through regularly scheduled departmental training sessions.

Staying committed to education also aids EMTs in developing their capacity to handle complex medical situations with greater expertise and confidence. This not only increases job satisfaction but also contributes to better patient outcomes. It is a responsibility shared by both the individual EMT seeking out opportunities for growth and by employers who should foster an environment encouraging continuous professional development.

Advancement Opportunities in EMS

For those who enter emergency medical services (EMS), there are numerous paths available for advancement. These range from achieving higher levels of certification (such as becoming an Advanced EMT or a Paramedic) to taking on supervisory or instructional roles.

The path to becoming a Paramedic offers one of the most significant steps up within EMS. This requires more comprehensive education and training which delves deeper into anatomy and physiology, cardiology, medications, and other complex areas of prehospital care. The elevated knowledge base and skill set allow paramedics to perform more advanced procedures than their Basic EMT counterparts, leading to increased autonomy on the scene and a broader scope of practice.

Opportunities outside of direct patient care also exist within EMS systems. Becoming an EMS educator or joining management ranks offers ways to contribute to field development while continuing to grow professionally. Educators can shape future generations of EMTs through program development or direct instruction, while those in managerial roles can influence operational protocols and policies.

In addition to formal promotions within a service's hierarchy, furthering education by obtaining degrees in emergency management or public health can open doors to roles within government agencies or private sector organizations focused on disaster response or health policy.

Regardless of the specific path chosen for advancement within EMS, dedication to ongoing education is paramount. Upgrading skills not only elevates an individual's ability to provide care but also enhances their leadership potential among peers. Medical emergencies will continue to present new challenges; thus, the commitment of each provider to grow professionally underpins the effectiveness and resilience of the entire EMS system.

Continuing education remains central both personally for individual providers' growth and collectively for enhancing EMS services' capacity to save lives proficiently. The interconnectedness between personal professional growth and community health emphasizes that lifelong learning is not just a beneficial endeavor—it's paramount for those tasked with serving at the front lines of emergency care.

Joining Professional Organizations and Networks

Another critical step for EMTs aiming for continuous advancement is to join professional organizations and networks. These entities serve as a valuable resource for information dissemination, professional development opportunities, advocacy efforts, and networking. Membership in organizations such as the National Registry of Emergency Medical Technicians (NREMT) or the National Association of Emergency Medical Technicians (NAEMT) provides several benefits.

Professional organizations often offer their members access to educational resources that can contribute to recertification credits. They also keep members informed on changes in laws and regulations affecting EMS practitioners through newsletters and official statements. Moreover, through conferences, symposiums, and seminars conducted by such organizations, EMTs can learn from thought-leaders in EMS fields about emerging trends.

Networking is yet another perk offered by these bodies; it encourages engagement with peers from diverse regions and service types. Peer interaction expands an individual's understanding of varied approaches to similar emergencies across different settings – urban versus rural or small private companies versus large municipal services.

Members can exchange knowledge about best practices and innovations or even discuss common challenges faced on the ground. Such relationships can not only enhance an individual's career by opening up job prospects but also provide moral support in managing work-related stress.

Professional organizations may even offer mentorship programs matching newer EMBs with seasoned professionals who can guide them through early career stages or during transitions to more advanced roles.

CONCLUSION
YOUR EMT CERTIFICATION JOURNEY

A s you come to the end of this guide, take a moment to acknowledge the significant progress you've made in your quest for EMT certification. It is a considerable achievement to have gained the knowledge and skills that will enable you to make a real difference in people's lives. Your dedication and hard work have brought you to this pivotal point in your journey. The effort you've invested in understanding complex medical procedures, memorizing protocols, and mastering the practical skills necessary for emergency response is commendable. The road to becoming a certified EMT is not just about passing a test; it's about committing to a life of service. Emergency Medical Services (EMS) is a vital part of the healthcare system, one that requires continuous learning and adaptation. The landscape of emergency care is ever-evolving, with new techniques, technologies, and challenges emerging regularly. Your initial certification is just the beginning of a lifelong educational journey.

Your success on the certification exam will open doors to new opportunities and responsibilities. Remember that every call for help is an opportunity to touch lives positively. The trust that individuals place in your hands during their most vulnerable moments is sacred, and with it comes the responsibility to always give your best. Stay curious and proactive about gaining more knowledge as healthcare advances unfold. This can mean enrolling in additional courses, attending workshops, or keeping up-to-date with EMS research findings. Set goals for further certifications or specializations within EMS if that feels like a good move for your career.

Keeping your skills sharp also involves practical experience on the field. You will learn much from colleagues who have been responding to emergencies for years. Be open to feedback and willing to share what you know; collaboration saves lives in our field more than any other. Moreover, don't forget self-care; it's easy to prioritize others' well-being over your own as an EMT but maintaining physical fitness, mental health, and emotional resilience is essential – not only for your welfare but also for providing the best care possible.

This guide aimed at preparing you for success – not just on the test but as a competent, compassionate EMT dedicated to saving lives and serving communities. As we part ways with this study guide, we leave you with one last sentiment: *May you always find courage in moments of fear, strength when you feel weak, and light on those nights that seem unbearably dark – because someone's worst day could be their best because of your help.*

Made in the USA
Monee, IL
20 November 2024

70658851R00063